The **NEW GLUCOSE REVOLUTION** Low GI Guide to

the Metabolic Syndrome

and Your Heart

Other **NEW GLUCOSE REVOLUTION** Titles

The New Glucose Revolution: The Authoritative Guide to the Glycemic Index—the Dietary Solution for Lifelong Health

The Low GI Diet Revolution

The Low GI Diet Cookbook

The New Glucose Revolution Low GI Eating Made Easy

The New Glucose Revolution Life Plan

The New Glucose Revolution What Makes My Blood Glucose Go Up . . . and Down?

The New Glucose Revolution Guide to Living Well with PCOS

The New Glucose Revolution Shopper's Guide to GI Values 2006

The New Glucose Revolution Low GI Guide to Sugar and Energy

The New Glucose Revolution Low GI Guide to Losing Weight

The New Glucose Revolution Low GI Guide to Diabetes

The New Glucose Revolution Pocket Guide to Peak Performance

The New Glucose Revolution Pocket Guide to Healthy Kids

The New Glucose Revolution Pocket Guide to Childhood Diabetes

FORTHCOMING

The New Glucose Revolution Low GI Vegetarian Cookbook

The New Glucose Revolution Low GI Eating Made Easy for Kids

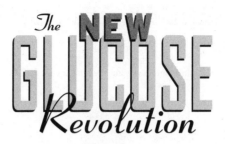

The **NEW**
GLUCOSE
Revolution

Low GI Guide to the

Metabolic
Syndrome

and Your Heart

The Only Authoritative Guide
to Using the Glycemic Index
for Better Heart Health

Dr. Jennie Brand-Miller
Kaye Foster-Powell
with Dr. Anthony Leeds

MARLOWE & COMPANY
NEW YORK

THE NEW GLUCOSE REVOLUTION LOW GI GUIDE TO THE
METABOLIC SYNDROME AND YOUR HEART:
The Only Authoritative Guide to Using the Glycemic Index for Better Heart Health

Published by
Marlowe & Company
An Imprint of Avalon Publishing Group, Incorporated
245 West 17th Street • 11th floor
New York, NY 10011

AVALON
publishing group incorporated

This edition is being published in somewhat different form in Australia in 2006 by
Hodder Australia, an imprint of Hachette Livre Australia Pty Ltd.
This edition is published by arrangement with Hachette Livre Australia Pty Ltd.

Library of Congress Cataloging-in-Publication Data
Brand Miller, Janette, 1952–
The new glucose revolution guide to the metabolic syndrome and your heart :
the only authoritative guide to using the glycemic index for better heart health /
Jennie Brand-Miller, Kaye Foster-Powell with Anthony Leeds.—2nd ed.
p. cm.—(New glucose revolution series)
Previous ed. had title: New glucose revolution pocket guide to
the metabolic syndrome and your heart.
Includes bibliographical references and index.
ISBN 1-56924-295-X (pbk.)
1. Metabolic syndrome—Handbooks, manuals, etc. 2. Glycemic index—
Handbooks, manuals, etc. 3. Heart—Diseases—Prevention—Handbooks, manuals, etc.
I. Brand Miller, Janette, 1952–. New glucose revolution pocket guide to the
metabolic syndrome and your heart. II. Foster-Powell, Kaye. III. Leeds, Anthony R.
IV. Title. V. Series.
RC662.4.B73 2006
616.1'205—dc22
2006007856

ISBN-13: 978-1-56924-295-7

9 8 7 6 5 4 3 2 1

Designed by Pauline Neuwirth, Neuwirth & Associates, Inc.

Printed in the United States of America

Contents

Introduction   1

PART ONE: Understanding Heart Disease   7
  Atherosclerosis   9
  What are the risk factors for heart disease?   11
  Smoking   12
  High blood pressure   13
  Diabetes and prediabetes (high blood glucose levels)   14
  High blood cholesterol   16
  CRP (C-reactive protein)   19
  Being overweight   19
  Being sedentary   24
  Understanding the metabolic syndrome   29
  What is insulin resistance?   31
  Test your heart knowledge   35

PART TWO: Understanding the GI   39
  The Glycemic Index—Today's Dietary Power Tool   41
  Why the rate of digestion has implications for your health   48
  Eating the low GI way   51

CONTENTS

"This For That"—substituting low GI for high GI foods 54

How does your diet rate? 56

Tips for making the change 61

PART THREE: 10 Steps to a Healthy Heart Diet 63

   1. Eat more whole grain breads and cereals 65

   2. Eat more legumes, including soybeans, chickpeas, and lentils 67

   3. Eat plenty of fruit and vegetables 69

   4. Eat more fish and seafood and boost your omega-3 intake 71

   5. Eat less saturated fat and replace bad fats with good fats 73

   6. Minimize your use of salt 75

   7. Moderate your alcohol intake 76

   8. Include nuts in your diet 77

   9. Use low-fat dairy and calcium-enriched soy products 78

  10. Eat lean red meats and skinless chicken 80

Putting the GI to work in your day 81

A week of heart-healthy low GI eating 84

More heart-healthy low GI meals 93

Mediterranean-style diets 96

Mediterranean-style menu 97

Heart-healthy Mediterranean meal ideas 98

Asian-style diets 102

Asian-style menu 104

Heart-healthy Asian-style meal ideas 106

PART FOUR: A to Z GI Tables 115

Reading sources and references 139

About the authors 143

Acknowledgments 145

Index 147

Introduction

LOW SATURATED FAT, LOW GI DIETS HELP PREVENT HEART DISEASE

*H*eart disease is the single biggest killer of Americans. Every 10 minutes, someone suffers a "cardiovascular event." So, what causes this deadly disease? Often it is the result of atherosclerosis, or hardening of the arteries, which develops slowly and can go virtually unnoticed until it produces problems such as angina or a heart attack. It's not just a cholesterol matter, however—we now know that inflammation of cells lining the blood vessels plays a key role.

Heart disease doesn't just happen. The signs will be there. One in two Americans over the age of 25 already has at least two features of a disease known as the metabolic syndrome, the insulin resistance syndrome, or Syndrome X. This is a collection of metabolic abnormalities including abdominal obesity and at least two of the following health problems—high blood pressure, high triglycerides, low levels of "good" HDL cholesterol, and diabetes or prediabetes—that increase the risk of atherosclerosis and heart attack.

These days, most people are well aware of the importance of cutting back on saturated fat and choosing the "good fats" for heart health. But did you know that being choosy about the type of carbohydrate you eat also helps prevent heart disease? This is because high blood glucose, the defining feature of diabetes and prediabetes, contributes to your risk of heart disease.

Research on the glycemic index (GI) shows that both the amount and type of carbohydrate you eat determines your blood glucose and insulin levels for many hours after you've eaten. We now know that the higher the GI of your diet, the greater your risk of heart disease.

The rate of carbohydrate digestion has important implications for everybody. High insulin levels resulting from a regular diet of high-GI carbs promotes high blood fats, high blood glucose, and high blood pressure—and increases your risk of heart attack.

A diet rich in slowly digested, low-GI carbs, on the other hand, along with regular exercise and the consumption of good fats, will reduce your risk of heart disease. By lowering your blood glucose after meals and reducing insulin levels you'll have:

- healthier blood vessels that are more elastic and dilate more easily
- "thinner" blood and improved blood flow
- more potential for weight loss and therefore less pressure on the heart
- better blood fats—more of the good cholesterol and less of the bad

What is the GI and why does it matter?

The glycemic index (GI) is simply a ranking of the carbohydrate in foods according to their immediate effect on blood glucose levels. It is defined by a standardized method of testing in human subjects and provides an easy and effective way to eat a healthy diet and control fluctuations in blood glucose.

- Carbohydrates that break down quickly during digestion have high GI values. Their blood glucose response is fast and high.
- Carbohydrates that break down slowly, releasing glucose gradually into the bloodstream, have a low GI.

One of the most important ways in which our diet differs from that of our ancestors is the speed of carbohydrate digestion and the resulting effect on blood glucose and insulin levels. Traditional diets all around the world contained slowly digested and absorbed carbohydrate—foods that we now know have a low GI value. By contrast, modern diets, with their highly processed, refined carbohydrates, are based on foods with a high GI value.

It's vital that people learn about the GI so they base their food choices on sound scientific evidence to help them choose the right amount and type of carbohydrate for their health and well-being.

In practical terms, you can reduce your risk of heart disease by eating more fruit and vegetables, whole grains, legumes (including beans, chickpeas, and lentils) and low-fat dairy foods.

Whatever your cultural background, you'll discover that eating the low GI way is filling, flexible, and sustainable. It suits the whole family. It's safe for adults and children, as well as for people with preexisting medical conditions such as heart disease, metabolic syndrome, diabetes, or polycystic ovarian syndrome (PCOS). When you are choosy about your carbohydrates, you'll find that:

- you will feel fuller for longer and will be less likely to overeat
- your insulin levels will be lower and you will store less fat
- over time, combined with regular daily exercise, a low GI diet will result in gradual weight loss

How to use this book

First we answer the pressing questions you may have about heart disease, the metabolic syndrome, the key causes and risk factors and what you can do to prevent them and take your heart health into your own hands.

In Part Two we show you how vitally important an understanding of the GI is for your heart health. We explain why choosing low-GI carbs—the slowly digested ones that produce smaller fluctuations in your blood glucose and insulin levels—are the secret to long-term health. And we show you how easy it is to make the change to a low GI diet.

Part Three describes our low GI heart-health diet, along with:

- practical tips to help you include more of the right sort of carbs in your diet and make the GI work for you throughout the day
- a week of low GI meal plans to suit people from a variety of backgrounds—American, Australian, Asian, Mediterranean, and Middle Eastern

Part Four explains how the GI is measured and lists the GI values of over 600 foods for easy reference when shopping or planning meals.

■

High glucose levels after eating have been shown to be an important predictor of cardiovascular disease. A low GI diet helps reduce blood glucose spikes.

■

PART ONE

Understanding Heart Disease

Most heart disease, whatever form it takes, is caused by atherosclerosis—thickening and hardening of the inside wall of the arteries through the slow build-up of fatty deposits (called plaques). This narrows the arteries and reduces blood flow.

ATHEROSCLEROSIS

*A*therosclerosis is a slow, progressive disease. Most people develop it so gradually that they live much of their lives blissfully unaware that it's even there. In fact, if it develops very slowly it may not cause any serious problems, even into great old age. But if you have other health problems such as high cholesterol or high blood glucose levels, it can develop faster and cause trouble sooner.

Although it's usually thought of as a "heart" disease, atherosclerosis can affect the arteries elsewhere in the body, including the brain, kidneys, arms, and legs. When it affects arteries to the heart and reduces blood flow, the heart muscle doesn't get enough oxygen for pumping blood, and eventually this causes pain, discomfort, and tightness in the chest (angina pectoris). There's a similar effect elsewhere in the body when blood flow is restricted by atherosclerosis: in the legs, it can cause muscle pains on exertion; in the brain, it can lead to a variety of problems from "funny feelings" to strokes.

An emergency occurs when a thrombosis (blood clot) forms over a patch of atherosclerosis in a major artery. This process can occur anywhere in the arterial system and can lead to a complete blockage of the blood flow. The consequences can range from a small heart attack to sudden death.

The likelihood of developing thrombosis is determined by the tendency of your blood to clot versus its natural ability to break down clots (fibrinolysis). A number of factors influence these counteracting tendencies and one is the level of glucose in your blood. Other factors include genes, exercise, and diet.

People who gradually develop atherosclerosis may slowly develop reduced heart function. For a while the heart will try to compensate for the problem, but eventually it begins to fail. Symptoms include shortness of breath, initially on exercise, and sometimes some swelling of the ankles. It can also lead to an abnormal heartbeat (palpitations).

Treating heart disease
When doctors detect signs of heart disease, they give two types of treatment.

- First, the effects of the disease are treated with drugs and/or with surgery to bypass blocked arteries.
- Secondly, the risk factors are treated to slow down further progression of heart disease. Treating risk factors after the disease has already developed is called "secondary prevention." In people who have not yet developed overt heart disease (such as those with the metabolic syndrome), treating the risk factors is called "primary prevention." Primary and secondary prevention includes diet and lifestyle advice on stopping smoking, the benefits of exercise, and a good diet for a healthy heart.

Many people find it hard to stay motivated to make big changes to diet and lifestyle if the effect of not following the advice is unlikely to matter for ten or more years. Long-term diet and lifestyle changes for heart health need to be positive ones: "I want to do this," not "they've told me to do this." Plenty of encouragement from friends and relatives helps.

■

TAKE ACTION AND REDUCE YOUR RISK
You can live a healthier, more active life by being positively involved in your own care through diet and lifestyle changes.

■

WHAT ARE THE RISK FACTORS FOR HEART DISEASE?

Your risk of developing heart disease is determined by things you cannot change, such as genetic (inherited) factors, and things you can do something about.

Risk factors you cannot change
- being male
- being older
- having a family history of heart disease
- being post-menopausal
- your ethnic background

Risk factors you can do something about
- smoking
- high blood pressure
- having diabetes or prediabetes (high glucose levels, but not as high as those in diabetes)
- having high blood cholesterol, high triglycerides, and low levels of the "good" (HDL) cholesterol

- having high CRP (C-reactive protein) levels (a marker of low-grade chronic inflammation somewhere in the body)
- being overweight or obese
- being sedentary

■

TAKE ACTION AND REDUCE YOUR RISK
Get regular medical checkups for blood pressure, diabetes, blood cholesterol, and blood glucose.

■

SMOKING

Smokers have more than twice the risk of heart attack as non-smokers and are much more likely to die if they suffer a heart attack. Smoking is also the most preventable risk factor for heart disease. Did you know:

- Smokers tend to eat fewer fruits and vegetables compared with nonsmokers and thus miss out on vital protective antioxidant plant compounds.
- Smokers tend to eat more fat and salt than non-smokers.

While these dietary differences may put the smoker at greater risk of heart disease, there is only one piece of advice for anyone who smokes: quit.

You can quit

There are plenty of options to help you kick the habit, from nicotine patches and gums to medication or even hypnosis. Talk to your doctor.

If you want to quit smoking, consider calling the quitline for help. Trained counselors can give you advice and assistance.

United States
National Network of Tobacco Cessation Quitlines
1-800-QUITNOW (1-800-784-8669)
Smoking cessation Web sites:
www.smokefree.gov
www.cdc.gov/tobacco
www.surgeongeneral.gov/tobacco

■

TAKE ACTION AND REDUCE YOUR RISK
If you smoke, quit.
Better yet, never start smoking at all!

■

HIGH BLOOD PRESSURE

High blood pressure is the most common heart disease risk factor. High blood pressure (hypertension) is harmful because it demands that your heart work harder and damages your arteries.

An artery is a muscular tube. Healthy arteries can change their size to control the flow of blood. High blood pressure causes changes in the walls of arteries which makes atherosclerosis more likely to develop. Blood clots can then form and the weakened blood vessels can easily develop a thrombosis or rupture and bleed.

Treatments for blood pressure have become more effective over the last 30 years, but it is only now becoming clear which types of treatment are also effective at reducing heart disease risk.

> **ABOUT THREE** in ten adults aged 25 and older have hypertension, defined as having blood pressure above 140/90 mm HG. This rises to one in two among older adults. An abnormal blood pressure is considered to be above 120/80.

■

TAKE ACTION AND REDUCE YOUR RISK
See your doctor. Today's blood pressure medications are effective, safe, and have fewer side effects.

■

DIABETES AND PREDIABETES (HIGH BLOOD GLUCOSE LEVEL)

Having diabetes is a risk factor for heart disease. Diabetes is caused by a lack of insulin—either the body does not produce enough, or the body "demands" more than normal because it has become insensitive to insulin. Diabetes and prediabetes (impaired glucose tolerance) cause inflammation and hardening of the arteries.

Be well, know your BGL

NORMAL RANGES for:

Fasting glucose	70–100 mg/dL
Glycated hemoglobin	4–6 %
Insulin	< 20 microunits/ml

High levels of glucose in the blood, even short-term spikes after a meal, can have many undesirable effects and are a predictor of future heart disease. Here's what happens . . .

A high level of glucose in the blood means:

- the cells lining the arteries take up excessive amounts of glucose
- highly reactive, charged particles called free radicals are formed which gradually destroy the machinery inside the cell, eventually causing cell death
- glucose adheres to cholesterol in the blood which promotes the formation of fatty plaque and prevents the body from breaking down the cholesterol
- higher levels of insulin, which in turn raises blood pressure and blood fats, while suppressing "good" (HDL) cholesterol levels

High insulin levels also increase the tendency for blood clots to form. This is why so much effort is put into helping people with diabetes achieve normal control of blood glucose levels. Even when cholesterol levels appear to be normal, other risk factors such as triglycerides can be highly abnormal.

But you don't need to have diabetes to be at risk—even moderately raised blood glucose levels before or after a meal have been associated with increased risk of heart disease in so-called normal, "healthy" people.

■

TAKE ACTION AND REDUCE YOUR RISK
Knowing your blood glucose level (BGL)
is as important as knowing your cholesterol level
or your blood pressure.
Ask your doctor.

■

HIGH BLOOD CHOLESTEROL

Cholesterol is vital for healthy cells. It is so important that our bodies make most of the cholesterol we need—about 1,000 mg per day. But in certain circumstances we make more than necessary. This causes the level of cholesterol in our blood to build up, and that's when we have a problem. When the body accumulates too much, cholesterol will be deposited on the walls of the arteries, which become bloated and damaged, and may become blocked.

Having high blood cholesterol is partly determined by our genes, which can "set" the cholesterol level slightly high and which we cannot change, and partly by lifestyle or dietary factors, which push it up further—which we *can* do something about.

A diet high in saturated fat is the biggest contributor. Diets recommended for lowering blood cholesterol are low in saturated fat, high in good carbohydrate, particularly whole grains, and high in fiber, including plant sterols—natural plant compounds that inhibit the absorption of cholesterol. Some vegetable oils are a rich source of these compounds, and new types of margarine may incorporate extra doses. While the quality of fat has been the traditional focus of dietary approaches, we are now learning that quality of carbohydrate can play a vital role in reducing the risk of heart disease.

Body weight also affects blood cholesterol levels. In most people, being overweight increases blood cholesterol and losing weight is very helpful.

There are some relatively rare genetic conditions in which particularly high blood cholesterol levels occur. People who have inherited these conditions need a rigorous cholesterol-lowering eating plan combined with drug treatment to reduce and control the risk of heart disease.

What about the good HDL cholesterol?

HDL (high-density lipoprotein) cholesterol seems to protect us against heart disease because it clears cholesterol from our arteries and aids its removal from our bodies. Having low levels of HDL in the blood is one of the most important markers of heart disease.

LDL cholesterol—the "bad" cholesterol

LDL (low-density lipoprotein) cholesterol does the most damage to blood vessels—it's a red flag for heart disease.

What about triglycerides?

The blood also contains triglycerides, another type of fat linked with increased risk of heart disease. Having too much triglyceride often goes hand in hand with having too little HDL cholesterol. People can inherit having excess levels of triglycerides, but it's most often associated with being overweight or obese.

Keeping your cholesterol in check

YOUR LEVELS of both cholesterol and triglyceride need to be checked by your doctor as part of an assessment of your risk of heart disease. The normal ranges are:

Cholesterol	< 200 mg/dL
Triglycerides	< 150 mg/dL
HDL cholesterol	< 60 mg/dL (different targets for men and women)
LDL cholesterol	< 100 mg/dl
Total cholesterol/HDL ratio	< 4.5

What about high-cholesterol foods?

Cholesterol in food is not the main cause of high blood cholesterol levels. The amount of cholesterol we obtain from food is generally much less than the amount our bodies make. Very few foods are high in cholesterol. They include brains, liver, kidney, egg yolk, and caviar.

Cholesterol absorption in the gut can vary between individuals—some people may be more sensitive to dietary cholesterol than others.

■

TAKE ACTION AND REDUCE YOUR RISK
Reducing your saturated fat intake can usually improve your blood cholesterol levels.
See your doctor.

■

CRP (C-REACTIVE PROTEIN)

Scientists have recently established that CRP in the blood is a powerful risk factor for heart disease. A measure of chronic low-grade inflammation anywhere in the body, it is indicative of the damaging effect of high glucose levels and other factors on the blood vessel walls.

In women, CRP levels may predict future risk of heart disease more effectively than cholesterol levels. Considering CRP and cholesterol levels together is a superior way for doctors to sort out those at greater risk.

Studies from Harvard have shown that CRP levels are higher in women consuming high GI/high glycemic load diets. That's one more good reason to choose low GI!

Inflammation— what does it mean?

INFLAMMATION IS the process by which the body responds to injury—anywhere in the body, whether it is gum disease, a bad cold, or a heart attack. Inflamed cells lining the blood vessels are the starting point for heart disease. C-reactive protein, a marker of general, low-grade inflammation, is now known to be a very good predictor of heart disease or stroke risk.

BEING OVERWEIGHT

Overweight and obese people are more likely to have high blood pressure and diabetes. They are also at increased risk of developing heart disease. Some of that increased risk is due to the high blood pressure, and the tendency to diabetes, but there is a separate, "independent" effect of the obesity.

When increased fatness develops, it can be distributed evenly all over the body or in and around the abdomen. The latter is strongly associated with heart disease. In fact, you can have "middle-age spread," a "beer gut," or a "pot belly" and still be within a normal weight range. But that extra fat around the middle is playing havoc with your metabolism. It's important to make every effort you can to lose a little weight and prevent further weight gain—especially if your extra weight is around your abdomen.

■

**Two in three men are overweight or obese.
Half of women are overweight or obese.**

■

Fat around the middle part of our body (abdominal fat) increases our risk of heart disease, high blood pressure, and diabetes. In contrast, fat on the lower part of the body, such as hips and thighs, doesn't carry the same health risk. Your body shape can be described according to your distribution of body fat as either an "apple" or a "pear" shape.

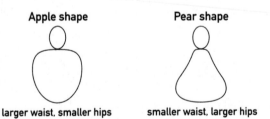

| Apple shape | Pear shape |
| larger waist, smaller hips | smaller waist, larger hips |

There are significant health benefits in reducing your waist measurement, particularly if you have an "apple" shape.

You can easily tell if you are an "apple" or a "pear." Simply place a tape measure around your waist and then your hips and see which is smaller. Ideally your waist is smaller than your hips. If it isn't, you're an apple!

Generally, the waist measurement for people 19 years and over should be:

- less than 40 inches for men
- less than 35 inches for women

Low GI foods and weight loss

If you are overweight, chances are you have looked at countless diet books, brochures, and magazines. New diets or miracle weight-loss solutions seem to appear weekly. At best, while you stick to it, a restrictive diet will reduce your calorie intake; at worst, it will change your body composition for the fatter.

The yo-yo pattern of weight gain and loss is all too familiar for serial dieters, and the overall effect of this pattern is often a weight increase of 4–7 pounds per year.

A healthy waist

THE INTERNATIONAL Diabetes Federation has published new criteria for defining the metabolic syndrome, reducing waist circumference thresholds to make it easier for doctors to identify people with the condition. (A person with metabolic syndrome will have abdominal obesity plus at least two of the following risk factors: high triglycerides, low HDL cholesterol, raised blood pressure, and/or raised blood glucose.)

continued

The cutoff waist measurements for people of Caucasian origin:
- Men   (37 inches)
- Women   (31.5 inches)

For people from South Asia and China:
- Men   (35.5 inches)
- Women   (31.5 inches)

For people from Japan:
- Men   (35.5 inches)
- Women   (33.5 inches)

For more information go to: www.idf.org/home/

Why? When you lose weight through severely restricting your food intake, you lose some of your body's muscle mass. Over the years this type of dieting will change your body composition to less muscle and proportionately more fat, making weight control increasingly difficult. Your body's engine will require less and less energy to keep it ticking. In fact, it is sad but true that 19 out of 20 people who lose weight by dieting will regain the lost weight.

It is not necessarily a matter of reducing how much you eat if you want to lose weight. Not all foods are equal. Research has shown that the type of food you give your body determines what it is going to burn and what it is going to store as body fat. We also know that certain foods are more satisfying to the appetite than others.

Low GI foods have two key advantages for people trying to lose weight:

- They fill you up and keep you satisfied for longer.
- They help you burn more body fat and less muscle.

■

TAKE ACTION AND REDUCE YOUR RISK
By eating right and exercising, you can lose weight
and reduce your risk of heart disease.

■

What's wrong with a low-carb diet?

ALTHOUGH LOW-CARB diets may help people lose weight, there are serious doubts about their long-term safety. They are often high in saturated fat—a risk factor for heart disease and cancer. They are often low in fruit and vegetables and therefore low in protective micronutrients. And in people with compromised kidney function, the need to filter more nitrogen can lead to kidney failure.

One reason for the popularity of low-carb diets is that initial loss is rapid. Within the first few days, the scales will be reading 4 to 7 pounds lower. The trouble is that some of that weight loss isn't body fat at all, but muscle mass and water.

People who have followed low-carbohydrate diets for any length of time observe that the rate of weight loss plateaus and they begin to feel tired and lethargic. That's not surprising, because the availability of glucose fuel to muscle is reduced. Strenuous exercise requires both fat and carbohydrate in the fuel mix. So, in the long term, low-carb diets may discourage people from physical exercise patterns that will help them keep their weight under control.

continued

Our advice is that the best diet for weight control is one you can stick to for life—one that includes your favorite foods and which accommodates your cultural and ethnic heritage. Choosing low GI foods will not only promote weight control, it will lower your blood glucose after meals, increase satiety, provide bulk and a rich supply of micronutrients.

Low GI diets are the happy compromise between a low-fat diet and a low-carb diet.

BEING SEDENTARY

These days it's all too easy to overeat. Highly refined, processed foods, convenience foods, and fast foods frequently lack fiber and conceal fat so that before we feel full, we have overdosed on calories.

It's even easier not to exercise. Many of us lead busy but sedentary, deskbound, commuting lives, exercising infrequently or not at all. People who aren't active or who don't exercise have higher rates of death from heart disease compared with people who perform even mild to moderate amounts of physical activity. Housework, gardening, or going for a walk on a regular basis can lower your risk of heart disease.

With food intake exceeding energy output on a regular basis, the result for too many of us is incremental weight gain.

How exercise helps
Regular physical activity can:

- help lower blood pressure
- cut heart attack and diabetes risk

- reduce insulin requirements if you have diabetes
- help you stop smoking
- control weight
- increase levels of "good" HDL cholesterol
- keep bones and joints strong
- reduce colon cancer risk
- improve mood
- ease depression
- increase stamina
- increase flexibility

It is meant for us all.

Exercise and activity speed up your metabolic rate (increasing the amount of energy you burn), which helps to balance your food intake—when you are active, your appetite is better "tuned" to energy output so you are less likely to eat more than you need. Exercise and activity also make your muscles more sensitive to insulin (you'll need less to get the job done) and increase the amount of fat you burn.

A low GI diet has the same effect. Low-GI foods reduce the amount of insulin you need, which makes fat easier to burn and harder to store. Since body fat is what you want to get rid of when you lose weight, exercise or activity in combination with a low GI diet makes a lot of sense.

The effect of exercise doesn't end when you stop moving. The more exercise you do, the more heat you produce as a by-product of metabolism. That extra heat production soaks up excess energy. People who exercise have higher metabolic rates and their bodies burn more calories per minute even when they are asleep!

Reduction in body weight takes time. So don't weigh yourself obsessively—use a tape measure around the waist instead. This is because, even after you've made changes in your exercise habits, your weight may not be any different, or not change very much, on the scales. This is particularly true for women, whose bodies tend to gain muscle and lose fat at the same time.

Improving cardiovascular fitness
Regular aerobic exercise that makes your heart beat faster and makes you breathe more deeply can improve your cardiovascular fitness. We need to accumulate at least 30 minutes each day of this level of exertion to maintain cardiovascular fitness.

■

TAKE ACTION AND REDUCE YOUR RISK

Some key factors to make exercise successful include:
- seeing a benefit for yourself (you can fit into your favorite jeans)
- enjoying what you do
- feeling that you can do it fairly well
- fitting in with your daily life
- being inexpensive and accessible

■

Exercise—we can't live without it.
All you have to do is accumulate
60 minutes of physical activity every day.

TO MAKE a real difference to your health and energy, physical activity has to be regular and some of it needs to be aerobic. But every little bit counts, so any extra you do is a step in the right direction. It can be hard to change the habits of a lifetime. That's why we suggest you "move it and lose it" with our "1,2,3 one step at a time, in your own time" approach.

1. Start with extra incidental activity

Incidental activity is the "exercise" you accumulate as part of your normal daily routines—making the bed, doing chores, walking to the bus stop or train station, running out for coffee, parking the car and walking to the stores or office. Think of extra incidental activity as an opportunity, not an inconvenience. See for yourself how "spending" five minutes here and there every day can add up to potential fat "savings" in the long term.

Take 5 minutes every day to:	Potential savings in pounds of fat*	
	In 1 year	In 5 years
Take the stairs instead of the elevator	8	40
Carry the groceries 500 feet to the car	3	11
Vacuum the living room	2	8
Walk 300 feet from the car to the office	1	6

* Figures based on a 154-pound person

2. Add time to move more

Walking keeps us fit, it's cheap and convenient, it gets us out and about, and it becomes even more important as we grow older. You can walk alone, or with friends. In fact, talking while you walk has other benefits: not only do our bodies produce calming hormones while we walk, but talking can be great therapy—and good for relationships and friendships, too.

How often? Try to walk every day. Ideally you

continued

should accumulate 30 minutes or more on most days of the week. The good news is you can do it in two 15-minute sessions or six 5-minute sessions. It doesn't matter.

How hard? You should be able to talk comfortably while you walk. Find a level that suits you. If you feel sore at first, don't worry; your body will adapt and the soreness will decrease. Stretching for 2 minutes before and after your walk will help minimize aches and pains.

How many steps? Thirty minutes of moderately paced walking is equivalent to 4,000 steps. Research has shown that every day we need to take about:

- 7,500 steps (45 minutes moderately paced walking) to maintain weight
- 10,000 steps (about 60 minutes briskly paced walking) to lose weight

3. Plus planned exercise

If you are ready to step up your fitness, making a commitment to a planned exercise program including aerobic, resistance, and flexibility/stretching exercises will give you the best results. The key is to find some activities you enjoy—and do them regularly. Just 30 minutes of moderate-intensity exercise each day can improve your health, reducing your risk of heart disease and type 2 diabetes. If you prefer you can break this into two 15-minute sessions or three 10-minute sessions. You'll still see the benefits.

Personal trainers

Working with a personal trainer can be a great way to improve your health and fitness and work toward your goals. A good trainer will design an exercise program tailored to your needs and fitness level as well as providing motivation and support. Many personal trainers now provide services for a reasonable rate, and you can choose to use a health club or train at home or outdoors. If cost is an issue, you could train with a group of three or four others with similar fitness levels, or you could just have a few sessions initially to get you started.

Before beginning a walking (or any exercise) program, see your doctor if you have:
- been inactive for some time
- a history of heart disease or chest pains
- diabetes
- high blood pressure

Or if you:
- weigh more than you should
- smoke

UNDERSTANDING THE METABOLIC SYNDROME

Surveys show that one in two adults over the age of 25 has at least two features of what is seen to be a "silent" disease: the metabolic syndrome, or insulin resistance syndrome. This syndrome, also called Syndrome X, is a collection of metabolic abnormalities that "silently" increase the risk of heart attack. The list of features is growing longer and longer, and the number of diseases linked to insulin resistance is growing.

People with metabolic syndrome are three times as likely to have a heart attack or stroke compared with people without the syndrome, and they have a fivefold greater risk of developing type 2 diabetes if it's not already present.

What is the metabolic syndrome?

The metabolic syndrome is a cluster of serious heart attack risk factors. In 2005, the International Diabetes Federation agreed on a new definition of metabolic syndrome to make it easier for doctors to identify people with this "cardiovascular time bomb." A person with metabolic syndrome will have central or abdominal obesity plus two of the following risk factors:

- high triglycerides
- low HDL cholesterol
- raised blood pressure
- raised blood glucose

The key to understanding metabolic syndrome is insulin resistance—tests on patients with the metabolic syndrome show that insulin resistance is very common. If your doctor has told you that you have high blood pressure and "a touch of sugar" (prediabetes or impaired glucose tolerance) then you probably have the insulin resistance syndrome.

The pancreas produces insulin

THE PANCREAS is a vital organ located near the stomach. Its function is to produce the hormone insulin. Carbohydrate stimulates the secretion of insulin more than any other component of food. The slow absorption of the carbohydrate in food means that the pancreas doesn't have to work so hard and produces less insulin. If the pancreas is overstimulated over a long period of time, however, it may become "exhausted," and type 2 diabetes may develop in genetically susceptible individuals. Even without diabetes, high insulin levels are undesirable because they increase the risk of heart disease.

■

TAKE ACTION AND REDUCE YOUR RISK

- Increase your physical activity
- Make sure your diet is low in saturated fat and low GI

■

WHAT IS INSULIN RESISTANCE?

Insulin resistance means that your body is insensitive, or "partially deaf," to insulin. The organs and tissues that ought to respond to even a small rise in insulin remain unresponsive. So your body tries harder by secreting more insulin to achieve the same effect. This is why high insulin levels are central to insulin resistance. You probably have insulin resistance if you have two or more of the following:

- high blood pressure
- low HDL cholesterol levels
- high waist circumference
- high uric acid levels in the blood
- prediabetes
- fasting glucose greater than 108 mg/dL

- post-glucose load greater than 140 mg/dL
- high triglycerides

Chances are your total cholesterol levels are within the normal range. You might also be of average weight but your waist circumference is high (more than 31.5 inches in women; more than 37 inches in men), indicating excessive fat around the abdomen.

But the red flag is that your blood glucose and insulin levels after eating remain high. Resistance to the action of insulin is thought to underlie and unite all the features of this cluster of metabolic abnormalities.

Why is insulin resistance so common?

Both genes and environment play a role. People of Asian and African-American origin and the descendants of the original inhabitants of Australia and North and South America appear to be more insulin resistant than those of Caucasian extraction, even when they are young and lean. But regardless of ethnic background, insulin resistance develops as we age, probably because as we grow older we gain excessive fat, become less active, and lose some of our muscle mass.

Diets with too much fat, especially saturated fat, and too little carbohydrate can make us more insulin resistant. If carbohydrate intake is high, eating high GI foods can worsen preexisting insulin resistance.

Why is insulin resistance a big deal?

The higher your insulin levels, the more carbohydrate you burn at the expense of fat. This is because insulin has two powerful actions: one is to "open the gates" so that glucose can flood into the cells and be used as the source of energy.

The second is to inhibit the release of fat from fat stores. The burning of glucose also reduces the burning of fat, and vice versa.

These actions persist even in the face of insulin resistance because the body overcomes the extra hurdle by simply pumping more insulin into the blood. Unfortunately, the level that finally drives glucose into the cells is two to ten times more than normal, encouraging fat storage instead of fat burning.

If insulin is high all day long, as it is in insulin-resistant and overweight people, then the cells are constantly forced to use glucose as their fuel source, drawing it from either the blood or stored glycogen. Blood glucose therefore swings from low to high and back again, playing havoc with appetite and triggering the release of stress hormones. The meager stores of carbohydrate in the liver and muscles also undergo major fluctuations over the course of the day.

When we don't get much chance to use fat as a source of fuel, fat stores accumulate wherever they can:

- inside the muscle cells (a sign of insulin resistance)
- in the blood (this is called high triglycerides, or TG, and is often seen in people with diabetes or the metabolic syndrome)
- in the liver (nonalcoholic fatty liver, or NAFL)
- around the waist (the proverbial pot belly)

Insulin resistance gradually lays the foundations of a heart attack and other health problems, such as stroke, polycystic ovarian syndrome (PCOS), fatty liver, acne, and cognitive impairment.

Research shows that low GI diets not only improve
blood glucose in people with diabetes, but also
improve the sensitivity of the body to insulin.

■

How can the GI help?

In a recent study, patients with serious disease of the
coronary arteries were given either low or high GI
diets before surgery for coronary bypass grafts. They
were given blood tests before their diets and just
before surgery, and at surgery small pieces of fat tissue were removed for testing.

The tests on the fat showed that the low GI diets
made the tissues of these "insulin insensitive"
patients more sensitive—in fact, they were back in the
same range as normal "control" patients after just a
few weeks on the low GI diet.

In another study, a group of women in their thirties
were divided into those who did and those who did not
have a family history of heart disease—and had not
yet developed the condition. They had blood tests followed by low or high GI diets for four weeks, after
which they had further blood tests. When they had
surgery (for conditions unrelated to heart disease),
pieces of fat were again removed and tested for
insulin sensitivity.

The young women with a family history of heart disease were insensitive to insulin originally (those without the family history of heart disease were normal),

but after four weeks on the low GI diet their insulin sensitivity was back within the normal range.

In both studies the diets were designed to try to ensure that all the other variables (total energy, total carbohydrates) were not different, so that the change in insulin sensitivity was likely to have been due to the low GI diet rather than any other factor.

TEST YOUR HEART KNOWLEDGE

Try this quick quiz on diet and heart disease to test your knowledge. Answer true or false to the following:

1. All vegetable oils are low in saturated fat.	T/F
2. Butter contains more fat than margarine.	T/F
3. Americans eat more fat now than they did 10 years ago.	T/F
4. Eggs should be avoided on a low-fat, cholesterol-lowering diet.	T/F
5. Moderate consumption of alcohol increases your risk of heart attack.	T/F
6. Olive oil has the lowest fat content of any oil.	T/F
7. A cup of milk contains less fat than two squares of chocolate.	T/F
8. Nuts will raise cholesterol levels.	T/F
9. Pasta makes you fat.	T/F
10. Cod liver oil will lower cholesterol levels.	T/F

The answer to each of the preceding questions is false. Here's why . . .

1. Contrary to popular belief, not all vegetable oils are low in saturated fat. Two primary exceptions are coconut oil and palm or palm kernel oil. Both these oils (which may appear on a food label simply as "vegetable oil") are highly saturated. Palm oil is used widely in commercial cakes, biscuits, pastries, and fried foods.

2. Butter and margarine contain similar levels of fat (around 85–90 percent). There is a difference in the types of fats which predominate, however, butter being about 60 percent saturated fat and unsaturated margarines being less than 30 percent saturated fat.

3. Americans are eating less fat now than they did 10 years ago. In 1988, we ate 35 percent of our energy in the form of fat. Now we are down to 32 percent, but we still have a way to go to achieve the target level of 30 percent. Plus, these are average figures, so many of us are still eating far too much fat.

4. Eggs are a source of cholesterol, but dietary cholesterol tends to raise blood cholesterol levels only when the background diet is high in fat. One egg contains only about 5 grams of fat, of which only 2 grams is saturated.

5. Moderate amounts of alcohol (e.g. 2 standard drinks per day) appear to reduce the risk of heart attack. Amounts in excess (3 or more) are harmful to health.

6. There is no such thing as low-fat oil. Oil is fat in a liquid form, its fat content being 100 percent. Olive oil is a suitable choice of oils, containing only 15 percent saturated fat. Mediterranean populations, whose major source of fat is olive oil, have low levels of heart disease.

7. A cup (8 fluid ounces) of full cream milk contains 10 grams of fat. Compare this to about 4 grams contained in two small squares of chocolate!

8. Nuts have been found to be protective against heart disease. While most nuts are high in fat, much of the fat they contain is of the "good" monounsaturated and polyunsaturated types.

9. This myth has been around for years. Pasta is, in fact, a low-GI food. Eaten with a tomato-based sauce, some protein and lots of vegetables, it is the perfect "dieter's" meal. Just go easy on the Parmesan cheese and cream sauces!

10. Cod liver oil does not lower cholesterol levels. Furthermore, it is extremely rich in vitamins A and D and should not be taken in large doses because of the danger of vitamin A toxicity.

PART TWO

Understanding the GI

What we know
today is that not all carbs
are created equal. In fact, they
can behave quite differently in our
bodies. The glycemic index, or GI,
is how we describe this difference,
ranking carbs (sugars and
starches) according to
their effect on blood
glucose levels.

THE GLYCEMIC INDEX—
TODAY'S DIETARY POWER TOOL

After testing hundreds of foods around the world, scientists have found that foods with a low GI will have less of an effect on blood glucose levels than foods with a high GI. High-GI foods cause spikes in glucose levels whereas low-GI foods encourage gentle rises and falls.

Switching to eating mainly low-GI carbs that slowly trickle glucose into your blood stream keeps your energy levels perfectly balanced and means you will feel fuller for longer between meals. The idea is to replace refined carbs such as white bread, sugary sweets, and puffed cereal products with less processed carbs such as whole grain bread, pasta, beans, fruit, and vegetables.

Choosing low-GI carbs will not only promote weight control, it will reduce blood glucose and insulin levels throughout the day, increase your sense of feeling full and satisfied, and provide bulk and a rich supply of micronutrients including zinc, calcium, and magnesium.

■

Research has shown that the type of carbohydrate we eat may have as much influence on our risk of heart disease as the type of fat.

■

Some key facts about carbs

CARBOHYDRATE IS a vital source of energy found in all plants and foods that come from plants, such as fruit, vegetables, cereals, and grains. The simplest form of carbohydrate is glucose, which is:

- a universal fuel for our bodies
- the only fuel source for our brain, red blood cells, and a growing fetus
- the main source of energy for our muscles during strenuous exercise

Our bodies rev on carbs. When we eat foods such as bread, cereals, and fruit, our body converts them into a sugar called glucose during digestion. It is this glucose that is absorbed from our intestine and becomes the fuel that circulates in our bloodstream. As the level of blood glucose rises after you have eaten a meal, your pancreas gets the message to release a powerful hormone called insulin. Insulin's job is to drive glucose out of the blood and into the cells. Once inside, glucose will be channeled into various pathways simultaneously—it will be used as an immediate source of energy, or converted to glycogen (a storage form of glucose), or, in exceptional circumstances, converted into fat. So insulin turns on glucose uptake and storage and turns off fat burning. For this reason, lowering insulin levels is one of the secrets to lifelong health. However, cutting carbs out all together is not the answer.

What exactly is the GI?

The glycemic index, or GI, is a ranking of carbohydrate quality describing how the carbohydrates in individual foods affect blood glucose levels. Foods with a high GI value contain carbohydrates that cause a dramatic rise in blood glucose levels, while foods with a low GI value contain carbohydrates with much less impact.

To make a fair comparison, all foods are compared with a reference food—pure glucose—and are tested in equivalent carbohydrate amounts.

- Carbohydrates that break down quickly during digestion have high GI values. Their blood glucose response is fast and high.
- Carbohydrates that break down slowly, releasing glucose gradually into the bloodstream, have a low GI.

Today we know the GI of hundreds of different food items that have been tested in people following the standardized method. We have included more than 600 GI values in the tables at the back of this book. For more detailed information consult www.glycemicindex.com.

■

The GI is a measure of how fast carbohydrates hit the bloodstream. It compares carbohydrates weight for weight, gram for gram.

■

What gives one food a high GI and another a low one?

The following table summarizes the results of the most recent scientific research on the various factors that influence the GI value of a food. The key message is that the physical state of the starch in a food is by far the most important factor influencing its GI value. That's why the advances in food processing over the past 200 years have had such a profound effect on the overall GI values of the carbohydrates we eat.

FACTORS THAT INFLUENCE THE GI VALUE OF A FOOD

FACTOR	MECHANISM	EXAMPLES OF FOOD WHERE THE EFFECT IS SEEN
Starch gelatinization	The less gelatinized (swollen) the starch, the slower the rate of digestion.	Al dente spaghetti and oatmeal have less gelatinized starch.
Physical entrapment	The fibrous coat around beans and seeds and plant cell walls acts as a physical barrier, slowing down access of enzymes to the starch inside.	Pumpernickel and grainy breads, legumes and barley.
High amylose to amylopectin ratio*	The more amylose a food contains, the less water the starch will absorb and the slower its rate of digestion.	Basmati rice and legumes contain more amylose than other cereals.
Particle size	The smaller the particle size, the easier it is for water and enzymes to penetrate (the surface area is relatively higher).	Finely milled flours have high GI values. Stone-ground flours have larger particles and lower GIs.

* Amylose and amylopectin are two different types of starch. Both are found in foods, but the ratio varies.

FACTOR	MECHANISM	EXAMPLES OF FOOD WHERE THE EFFECT IS SEEN
Viscosity of fiber	Viscous, soluble fibers increase the viscosity of the intestinal contents and this slows down the interaction between the starch and the enzymes.	Finely milled whole wheat and rye flours have fast rates of digestion and absorption because the fiber is not viscous. Rolled oats, beans, lentils, and apples, on the other hand, are good examples.
Sugar	The digestion of sugar produces only half as many glucose molecules as the same amount of starch (the other half is fructose). The presence of sugar also restricts gelatinization of the starch by binding water and reducing the amount of "available" water.	Oatmeal cookies and some breakfast cereals (Kellogg's Frosted Flakes) that are high in sugar have relatively low GI values.
Acidity	Acids in food slow down stomach emptying, thereby slowing the rate at which starch can be digested.	Vinegar, lemon juice, lime juice, some salad dressings, pickled vegetables and sourdough bread.
Fat	Fat slows down the rate of stomach emptying, thereby slowing the digestion of starch.	Potato chips have a lower GI value than boiled white potatoes.

The key to understanding GI is the rate of digestion

Foods containing carbohydrates that break down quickly during digestion have the highest GI value. The blood glucose response is fast and high (in other words, the amount of glucose in the bloodstream increases rapidly). On the other hand, foods containing carbohydrates that break down slowly, releasing glucose gradually into the bloodstream, have low GI values.

For most people, those foods with low GI values have advantages over those with high GI values. This is especially true for people trying to prevent the onset of the metabolic syndrome and atherosclerosis.

The higher the GI, the higher the blood glucose levels after consumption of the food. Instant white rice (GI 87) and baked potatoes (GI 85) have very high GIs, meaning their effect on blood glucose levels is almost as high as that of an equal amount of pure glucose (yes, you read it correctly!)

The benefits of understanding the GI

UNDERSTANDING THE GI will help you base your food choices on sound scientific evidence by:

- helping you choose the right amount and type of carbohydrate for your health and well-being
- providing an easy and effective way to eat a healthy diet and control fluctuations in blood glucose

UNDERSTANDING THE GI

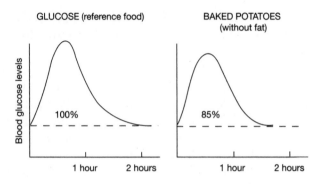

Figure 1

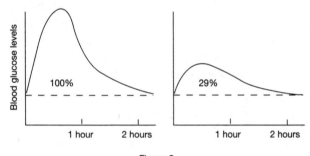

Figure 2

Figure 1 shows the blood glucose response to potatoes compared with pure glucose. Foods with a low GI (like lentils at 29) show a flatter blood glucose response when eaten, as shown in Figure 2. The peak blood glucose level is lower and the return to baseline levels is slower than with a high-GI food.

■

Low GI = 55 or less
Medium GI = 56 to 69
High GI = 70 or more

■

WHY THE RATE OF DIGESTION HAS IMPLICATIONS FOR YOUR HEALTH

The type of carbohydrate you eat determines your body's blood glucose response and also determines the levels of insulin in your blood for many hours after eating. High insulin levels caused by eating foods with a high GI are undesirable. In the long term, they promote high blood fats, high blood glucose, high blood pressure, and increase the risk of heart attack. Because of this, the GI of your diet is significant in the long-term prevention of heart disease and may be equally important in the diets of people who already have heart disease.

Low GI diets also reduce total blood cholesterol and "bad" low-density lipoprotein (LDL) cholesterol in people with undesirably high levels. Lower levels of total cholesterol and LDL cholesterol are associated with a lower risk of heart disease.

Large-scale studies of the diets and health of thousands of people have shown that "good" high-density lipoprotein (HDL) cholesterol levels are correlated with the GI and glycemic load of the diet. Those of us who choose the lowest GI diets have the highest and best levels of HDL. The presence of HDL cholesterol is a sign of cholesterol being taken away from arteries, so the higher the levels the better. High HDL cholesterol is the best predictor of a lower risk of heart disease; a low level of HDL is one of the key features of the metabolic syndrome.

Furthermore, research studies in people with diabetes have shown that low GI diets reduce triglycerides in the blood, a factor strongly linked to the metabolic syndrome.

Lastly, low GI diets have been shown to improve insulin sensitivity in people at high risk of heart disease, thereby helping to reduce the rise in blood glucose and insulin levels after normal meals.

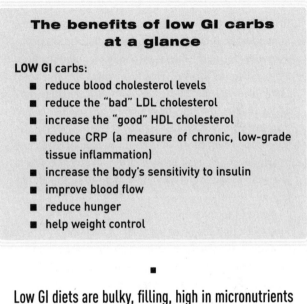

The benefits of low GI carbs at a glance

LOW GI carbs:

- reduce blood cholesterol levels
- reduce the "bad" LDL cholesterol
- increase the "good" HDL cholesterol
- reduce CRP (a measure of chronic, low-grade tissue inflammation)
- increase the body's sensitivity to insulin
- improve blood flow
- reduce hunger
- help weight control

■

Low GI diets are bulky, filling, high in micronutrients and good fats, and they help weight control.
The risk factors for heart disease are improved by eating a low GI diet.

■

GI and heart disease:
the weight of evidence

ONE STUDY that has provided the strongest evidence in support of the role of GI in heart disease was conducted by Harvard University and is commonly known as the "Nurses' Study." This is an ongoing, long-term study of over 100,000 nurses who provide their personal health and diet information to researchers at Harvard School of Public Health every few years. The study found that those who ate more high GI foods had nearly twice the risk of having a heart attack over a ten-year period of follow-up, compared to those eating low GI diets.

One of the most important findings of the Nurses' Study was that the increased risk associated with high GI diets was largely seen in those with a body mass index (BMI) over 23. There was no increased risk in those under 23. The great majority of adults, however, have a BMI greater than 23; indeed, a BMI of 23–25 is considered normal weight. The implication, therefore, is that the insulin resistance that comes with increasing weight is an integral part of the disease process.

To calculate your body mass index (BMI) divide your weight in pounds by your height in inches, squared, then multiply by 705.

$$BMI = Weight\ (pounds) \div Height\ (inches)^2 \times 705$$

So, if you are very lean and insulin sensitive, high GI diets won't make you more prone to heart attack. This might explain why traditional-living Asian populations, such as the Chinese, who eat high GI rice as a staple food, do not show increased risk of heart disease. Their low BMI and their high level of physical activity work together to keep them insulin-sensitive and extremely carbohydrate-tolerant.

EATING THE LOW GI WAY

The basic technique for eating the low GI way is simply "this for that": swapping high GI carbs with low GI carbs. This could mean eating muesli at breakfast instead of wheat flakes, a low GI grainy-bread instead of a processed white or whole wheat bread, or a sparkling apple juice in place of a soft drink.

■

You don't need to count numbers or do any sort of mental arithmetic to make sure you are eating a healthy, low GI diet.

■

Here are some points to keep in mind when putting the GI into practice.

The GI only relates to carbohydrate-rich foods

The foods we eat contain three main nutrients—protein, carbohydrate, and fat. Some foods, such as meat, are high in protein, while bread is high in carbohydrate and butter is high in fat. We need to eat a variety of foods (in varying proportions) to provide all three nutrients, but the GI only applies to high carbohydrate foods. This means bread, rice, pasta, potato, and cereals have GI values, but foods without much (if any) carbohydrate—such as meat, fish, eggs, and cheese—don't. There are other nutritional qualities to consider when you're choosing these foods.

The GI is not intended to be used in isolation

The GI of a food does not make it good or bad for us. High GI foods like potatoes and whole wheat bread still make valuable nutritional contributions to our diet. And low GI foods like pastry that are high in saturated fat are no better for us because of their low GI. The nutritional benefits of different foods are many and varied, and we suggest you base your diet on a wide variety of foods which are low in salt and saturated fat, high in fiber and have a low GI.

You don't need to avoid all high GI foods

There is no need to eat only low GI foods. While you will benefit from eating low GI carbs at each meal, this doesn't have to be at the exclusion of all others. A meal consisting of a high GI food such as potato with a lower GI food such as corn will result in a medium GI overall.

You don't need to add up the GI each day

In some of our early books we included sample menus and calculated an estimated GI for the day. As our understanding of the GI grew and we talked to our clients and heard from our readers, we realized how unnecessary and misleading this was. The GI value of a food can be altered by the way it is processed or cooked, so we don't believe it is possible to calculate a precise GI value for recipes or to predict the GI of a menu for the whole day. That's why we now prefer simply to categorize recipes and menus as low, medium, or high

GI. We have also seen the benefits people gain by simply substituting low for high GI foods in their everyday meals and snacks without more complicated dietary changes.

There's no point wondering about the GI of meat, chicken, fish, eggs, and cheese

These foods don't have one. It is not scientifically possible to measure a GI value for foods that contain negligible (or no) carbohydrate. But these foods are part of a healthy balanced diet and we're asked about them all the time, so we have included them in our tables with this symbol * (star) so that you know the GI is not relevant.

You don't need to be pedantic about GI values

Whether a food's GI is 56 or 64 isn't biologically relevant. Normal day-to-day variation in the human body could obscure the difference in these values. Generally a variation of more than 10 could be considered significant.

GL (glycemic load) vs GI—what's all the fuss about?

Your blood glucose rises and falls when you eat a meal containing carbohydrate. How high it rises and how long it remains high depends on the quality of the carbohydrate as well as the quantity of carbohydrate in your meal. Researchers at Harvard University came up with a term that combines these two factors—glycemic load (GL).

When comparing foods, should you use the GL instead of GI?

More often than not it's low GI rather than low GL that predicts good health outcomes. When you choose low GI carbs, you're eating healthier, high-quality carbs and you're more likely to be eating the right quantity of carbohydrate, too. Following the low GL path could mean your diet is low in carbs and full of the wrong sorts of fats such as butter and fatty meats.

■

Don't get carried away with GL.
It doesn't distinguish between low carb and slow carb.

■

What's all the fuss about? Some carb-rich foods such as pasta have a low GI but could have a high GL if the serving size is large. Portion sizes count. And while it's true a small number of high GI foods, such as watermelon, parsnips, and pumpkin, have a low GL, we don't want you to restrict any fruit or vegetable other than potato.

There's no denying it is easy to overeat some foods. This is where low GI foods are star performers—the foods with the lowest GI values also have the best fill-up factor.

■

Use GI to identify the best carbohydrate choices.
Take care with portion size to control the
overall GL of your diet.

■

"THIS FOR THAT"—SUBSTITUTING
LOW GI FOR HIGH GI FOODS

Simply substituting high GI foods with low GI alternatives will give your overall diet a lower GI and deliver the benefits of low GI eating. Here's how you can put slow carbs to work in your day by cutting back consumption of high GI foods and replacing them with alternatives that are just as tasty.

If you are currently eating this (high GI) food . . .	. . . choose this (low GI) alternative instead
Cookies	A slice of whole grain bread or toast with jam, fruit spread, or Nutella®
Smooth textured breads such as soft white or whole wheat, rolls, scones	Dense breads with whole grains, whole grain and stoneground flour, and sourdough; look for the GI symbol
Breakfast cereals—most commercial, processed cereals including corn flakes, rice crispies, cereal "biscuits"	Traditional rolled oats, muesli and the commercial low GI brands listed in the tables; look for the GI symbol
Cakes and pastries	Raisin toast, fruited breads, and fruited buns are healthier baked options; yogurts and low-fat pudding also make great snacks or desserts
Chips and other packaged snacks such as cheese curls, pretzels	Fresh grapes or cherries; dried fruit and nuts
Crackers	Crisp vegetable strips such as carrot, pepper, or celery
Doughnuts and croissants	Skim milk cappuccino or smoothie
French fries	Leave them out! Have salad or extra vegetables instead. Corn on the cob or coleslaw are better takeout options
Candy	Chocolate is lower GI but high in fat. Healthier options are nuts, raisins, dried apricots, and other dried fruits
Granola bars	Try a nut bar or dried fruit and nut mix; look for low GI labeling

If you are currently eating this (high GI) food . . .	. . . choose this (low GI) alternative instead
Potatoes	Prepare smaller amounts of potato and add some sweet corn; canned new potatoes are an easy and lower GI option; you can also try sweet potato, yam, taro, or baby new potatoes—or just replace with other low GI or no-GI vegetables
Rice, especially large servings of it in dishes such as risotto, nasi goreng, fried rice	Try basmati or Uncle Ben's converted long-grain rice, pearled barley, bulgur, quinoa, pasta, or noodles
Soft drink and fruit juice drink	Use a variety if you drink these often; fruit juice has a lower GI (but it is not a lower calorie option); water is best
Sugar	Moderate the quantity; consider 100% pure floral honey, apple juice, and fructose powder as alternatives

HOW DOES YOUR DIET RATE?

Reducing the GI of your diet will decrease insulin levels and increase the potential for fat burning. You can achieve an effective reduction in the GI by substituting at least one high GI carbohydrate choice at each meal with a low GI food. It's the carb foods you eat the most of that have the greatest impact—so check your intake in the following quiz.

What type of carbohydrate did you eat yesterday?

1. Recall the carbohydrate-rich foods you ate yesterday. Remember the snacks as well as the main meals!

2. Check the boxes below for the types of foods you
    ate.

HIGH GI	LOW GI

Starchy foods

HIGH GI	LOW GI
❏ Potato, including baked, mashed, steamed, boiled, and French fries ❏ Rice (arborio, quick-cooking, instant, jasmine)	❏ Sweet corn ❏ Baked beans ❏ Sweet potato ❏ Chickpeas ❏ Kidney beans, lentils ❏ Pasta ❏ Noodles ❏ Basmati, brown, or Uncle Ben's converted long-grain rice

Bread products

HIGH GI	LOW GI
❏ White bread ❏ Whole wheat bread ❏ Rolls ❏ Croissants ❏ Scones ❏ Bagels ❏ French bread	❏ Whole grain bread ❏ Fruited bread, raisin toast ❏ Sourdough bread ❏ Soy and flaxseed bread

Cereals

HIGH GI	LOW GI
❏ Cornflakes ❏ Rice Krispies ❏ Cocoa Krispies ❏ Puffed Wheat ❏ Weet-Bix™	❏ Special K ❏ Oatmeal ❏ Muesli ❏ All-Bran ❏ Frosted Flakes

Cookies

HIGH GI	LOW GI
❏ Water crackers ❏ Graham crackers ❏ Vanilla wafers ❏ Rice cakes ❏ Shortbread	❏ Rich Tea Cookie ❏ Oatmeal cookies

continued

HIGH GI	LOW GI
Snacks	
❏ Candy	❏ Dried apricots
❏ Muesli bars	❏ Prunes
❏ Pretzels	❏ Nuts
❏ Cheese curls	❏ Yogurt
	❏ Milk
	❏ Ice cream
Fruit	
❏ Watermelon	❏ Apples
❏ Dates	❏ Oranges
	❏ Bananas
	❏ Grapes
	❏ Kiwi fruit
	❏ Peaches, plums, apricots

3. Now add up the number of marks in each column of foods. The foods in the left column have a high GI. If most of your marks are in this column, you are eating a high GI diet. Consider altering some of your choices to include more of the foods from the column on the right.

Is your diet too high in fat?

Use this fat counter to tally up how much fat your diet contains. Circle all the foods that you could eat in a day, look at the serving size listed, and multiply the grams of fat up or down to match your serving size. For example, with milk, if you estimate you might consume 2 cups of regular milk in a day, this supplies you with 16 grams of fat.

Food	Fat content (grams)	How much did you eat?
Dairy Foods		
Milk, 1 cup		
Regular	8	
Reduced-fat 2 %	5	
Low-fat 1%	3	
Fat-free	0	
Yogurt, 8-ounce container		
Regular	6	
Low-fat	3	
Ice cream, 2 scoops (½ cup)		
Regular, vanilla	5	
Reduced-fat, vanilla	3	
Cheese		
Regular cheese, ¾-ounce slice	5	
Reduced-fat, 1-ounce slice	2	
Low-fat slices (per slice)	2	
Cottage cheese, 2 tablespoons	2	
Ricotta cheese, part skim, 2 tablespoons	2	
Cream/sour cream, 1 tablespoon		
Regular	3	
Reduced-fat	2	
Fats and oils		
Butter/margarine, 1 teaspoon	4	
Oil, any type, 1 tablespoon	14	
Cooking spray, per spray	1	
Mayonnaise, 1 tablespoon	11	
Salad dressing, 1 tablespoon	7	
Meat		
Beef		
Steak, 1 medium (6 ounces), fat trimmed	5	
Ground beef patty (6 ounces), cooked, drained	21	
Sausage, 1 thick, grilled (3 ounces)	13	
Top roast, 2 slices, lean only (3 ounces)	5	
Lamb		
Chop, grilled/BBQ, 2, fat trimmed	10	
Leg, roast meat, lean only, 2 slices (2 ounces)	6	
Loin chop, grilled/BBQ, 2, lean only	6	

continued

Food	Fat content (grams)	How much did you eat?
Pork		
Bacon, 1 slice, grilled	6	
Ham, 1 slice, leg, lean	1	
Butterfly steak, fat trimmed	3	
Leg, roast meat, 3 slices (3 ounces) lean only	6	
Large chop, fat trimmed	9	
Chicken		
Breast, skinless, 5 ounces	5	
Drumstick, skinless	5	
Thigh, skinless	8	
½ barbecue chicken (including skin)	17	
Fish		
Grilled fish, 1 average fillet	3	
Salmon, 2 ounces	5	
Fish sticks, 4 grilled	10	
Fish fillets, 2, breaded, commercial, oven baked		
Regular	20	
Light	16	
Snack foods		
Chocolate (1¾-ounce bar)	15	
Potato crisps (1¾ ounce)	15	
Corn chips (1¾ ounce)	18	
Peanuts, (1 ounces)	14	
French fries, medium serving	20	
Pizza, 2 slices, medium pizza	20	
Total		

How did you rate?

Less than 40 grams — Excellent. Between 30 and 40 grams of fat per day is an average range recommended for those trying to lose weight.

41–60 grams — Good. A fat intake in this range is recommended for most adult men and women.

| 61–80 grams | Acceptable, if you are very active, i.e., doing hard physical work (laboring) or athletic training. It is too much if you are trying to lose weight. |
| More than 80 grams | You're possibly eating too much fat, unless of course you are Superman or Superwoman! |

TIPS FOR MAKING THE CHANGE

Some people change their eating habits easily, but for the majority of us, change of any kind is difficult. Changing our diet is seldom just a matter of giving up certain foods. A healthy diet contains a wide variety of foods but we need to eat them in appropriate proportions. If you are considering changes to your diet, keep these guidelines in mind.

- Aim to make changes gradually.
- Attempt the easiest changes first.
- Break big goals into a number of smaller, more achievable goals.
- Accept lapses in your habits.
- If you feel you need some help, make an appointment to see a dietitian.

■

**Low saturated fat + low GI =
prevention of heart disease**

■

Find a good dietitian

REGISTERED DIETITIANS (RDs) have professionally recognized qualifications in human nutrition. They can provide specific advice tailored to your current eating habits and food preferences, and will work with you to set realistic and achievable goals. They will help you understand the relationship between food and health and guide you in making dietary choices that best suit your lifestyle. Dietitians practice as individual professionals and are available through most public hospitals and in private practice.

To find a dietitian:

Visit "Find a Dietitian" www.eatright.org
or call the American Dietetic Association
  at 1-800-877-1600

PART THREE

10 STEPS TO A HEALTHY HEART DIET

1. Eat more whole grain breads and cereals

2. Eat more legumes, including soybeans, chickpeas, and lentils

3. Eat plenty of fruit and vegetables

4. Eat more fish and seafood and boost your omega-3 intake

5. Eat less saturated fat and replace bad fats with good fats

6. Minimize your use of salt

7. Moderate your alcohol intake

8. Include nuts in your diet

9. Use low-fat dairy and calcium-enriched soy products

10. Eat lean red meats and skinless chicken

1. EAT MORE WHOLE GRAIN BREADS AND CEREAL

By "whole grain" we simply mean grains that are eaten in nature's packaging—or close to it: traditional rolled oats, cracked wheat, and pearl barley for example. The slow digestion and absorption of these foods will trickle fuel into your engine at a slower rate, keeping you satisfied for longer.

There are countless reasons to include more whole-cereal grains in your diet, but it's hard to go past the fact that because you are eating the whole grain, you get all the benefits of its vitamins, minerals, protein, dietary fiber, and protective antioxidants. Studies around the world show that eating plenty of whole grain cereals reduces the risk of certain types of cancer, heart disease, and type 2 diabetes.

A higher fiber intake, especially from whole-cereal grains, is linked to a lower risk of cancer of the large bowel, breast, stomach, and mouth. Eating these higher fiber foods can help you lose weight because they fill you up sooner and leave you feeling full for longer. They improve insulin sensitivity, too, and lower insulin levels.

We can still gain the benefit of whole grains in our diet today with foods such as:

- barley—e.g., pearl barley in soup, or in recipes such as barley risotto

- whole wheat or cracked wheat such as bulgur in tabbouleh
- rolled oats for breakfast as porridge or in muesli
- whole grain breads (with chewy grains and seeds)

Are you eating enough fiber? You need about 30 grams a day

MANY LOW GI foods are a good source of dietary fiber. Dietary fiber comes from plant foods—it is found in the outer bran layers of grains (corn, oats, wheat, and rice and in foods containing these grains), fruit and vegetables, and nuts and legumes (dried beans, peas, and lentils). There are two types—soluble and insoluble—and there is a difference.

Soluble fibers are the gel, gum, and viscous (jelly-like) components of apples, oats, and legumes. They are part of what gives these foods a low GI. Eating a diet rich in soluble fiber is a good way of maintaining a healthy heart, as soluble fiber helps to reduce cholesterol absorption. Foods rich in soluble fiber include fresh fruit and vegetables, legumes, and grain-based foods made from oats, barley, and psyllium.

Insoluble fibers are dry and branlike and are commonly known as roughage. All cereal grains and products made from them that retain the outer coat of the grain are sources of insoluble fiber, such as whole wheat bread and All-Bran, but not all foods containing insoluble fiber are low GI.

2. EAT MORE LEGUMES, INCLUDING SOYBEANS, CHICKPEAS, AND LENTILS

Look no further than legumes for a low GI food that is easy on the budget, versatile, filling, nutritious, and low in calories and fat. Legumes are high in fiber, too—both soluble and insoluble—and are packed with nutrients, providing a valuable source of protein, carbohydrate, B vitamins, folate, iron, zinc, and magnesium. Whether you buy dried beans, lentils, and chickpeas and cook them yourself at home, or opt for the very convenient, time-saving canned varieties, you are choosing one of nature's lowest GI foods.

A bean meal doesn't always have to be vegetarian—try using beans in place of grains or potatoes. You could serve a bean salsa with fish, or white bean purée with grilled meat. Butter beans can also make a delicious potato substitute.

Because they are high in protein, legumes are an ideal substitute for meat. Introduce them to your family gradually by incorporating them in meals with meat—as chili con carne or a filling for tacos or burritos, for example. You could also try:

- three-bean mix with a salad
- canned kidney beans in a bolognese sauce
- hummus dip or spread
- pea and ham soup
- potato bake with onions, beans, and lean bacon

The special benefits of soy

SOYBEANS AND soy products such as tofu and tempeh have been a staple part of Asian diets for thousands of years and are an excellent source of protein. They are also rich in fiber, iron, zinc, and vitamin B. They are lower in carbohydrate and higher in fat than other legumes, but the majority of the fat is polyunsaturated. Soy is also a rich source of phytochemicals.

Foods based on soybeans also have a beneficial role in our defense against heart disease. There are two components of soybeans with the potential to reduce heart disease risk: soy protein and antioxidant substances called isoflavones. Soy foods:

- improve blood fats, lowering the bad (LDL) cholesterol
- increase the good (HDL) cholesterol
- reduce the accumulation of cholesterol in blood vessels by decreasing LDL oxidation and thereby inflammation
- decrease the tendency to form blood clots

Studies suggest that one to two servings of soy protein-rich food each day may be sufficient to provide long-term health benefits. Just one cup of soy milk constitutes a serving and can be used as a nutritionally balanced replacement for dairy milk, providing it is low-fat and calcium enriched. Try:

- soy milk on your breakfast cereal
- a soy banana smoothie
- a soy yogurt for a snack

3. EAT PLENTY OF FRUIT AND VEGETABLES

High in fiber and low in fat (apart from olives and avocado, which contain some "good" fats), fruit and vegetables play a central role in a healthy-heart diet. Increased consumption of fruit and vegetables is associated with a lower incidence of diseases such as cancer, cardiovascular disease and other age-related diseases.

Fruit and vegetables are bursting with nutrients that will give you a glow of good health, such as:

- Beta-carotene—the plant precursor of vitamin A, used to maintain healthy skin and eyes. A diet rich in beta-carotene may even lessen skin damage caused by UV rays. Apricots, peaches, mangoes, carrots, broccoli, and sweet potato are particularly rich in beta-carotene.
- Vitamin C—nature's water-soluble antioxidant. Antioxidants are a bit like your personal bodyguard, protecting your cells from the damage that occurs as a natural part of aging and from pollutants in the environment. Guava, pepper, orange, kiwi fruit, and cantaloupe are especially rich in vitamin C.
- Anthocyanins—the purple and red pigments in blueberries, peppers, beets, and eggplant which also function as antioxidants, minimizing the damage to cell membranes that occurs with aging.

Get into the fruit and vegetable habit
- Make sure your main meal includes vegetables. Pile your plate high with leafy green and salad "free" foods that are full of fiber, essential nutrients and protective antioxidants that will fill you up without adding extra calories.

- When eating out, order a side salad with your meal (and pass on the fries!)
- Try a new vegetable each week.
- Take an apple and a banana to work.
- Make a habit of eating some fruit at home when you relax in the evening.
- Consider fresh, canned, dried, and juiced fruit as sources of fruit for your diet.
- Chop fresh pineapple or melon into large chunks and keep on hand in the refrigerator for snacks during the day.
- Serve a fruit platter for the family to share after a meal as dessert.

What about potatoes?

BOILED, MASHED, baked, or fried, everybody loves potatoes. However, we now know that the GI value of potatoes can differ significantly depending on variety and cooking method (GI 56 to 89), according to University of Toronto researchers reporting recently in the *Journal of the American Dietetic Association*. Their study found that precooking and reheating potatoes, or consuming cold cooked potatoes (such as potato salad), reduces the glycemic response. The highest GI values were found in potatoes that were freshly cooked and in instant mashed potatoes.

In our testing so far in Australia, the only potatoes to make the medium GI range are tiny, new canned ones (GI 65).

There's no need to avoid potatoes altogether just because they may have a high GI. They are fat free (when you don't fry them), nutrient rich, and filling. Not every food you eat has to have a low GI. So enjoy them, but in moderation. Try steaming small new potatoes (with their skin for added nutrients), or bake a russet potato and add a tasty topping based on beans, chickpeas, or corn kernels. Add variety to meals and occasionally replace potatoes with sweet corn, sweet potato or yams, or serve pasta, noodles, basmati rice, or legumes.

4. EAT MORE FISH AND SEAFOOD AND BOOST YOUR OMEGA-3 INTAKE

Increased fish consumption is linked to a reduced risk of heart disease, improvements in mood, lower rates of depression, better blood fat levels, and enhanced immunity. Just one serving of fish a week may reduce the risk of a fatal heart attack by 40 percent!

The likely protective components of fish are the very long chain omega-3 fatty acids. Our bodies only make small amounts of these unique fatty acids, so we rely on dietary sources, especially fish and seafood, for them. They can reduce inflammation in the body, iron out irregularity in heart beat, reduce blood fat levels and might play a valuable role in treating depression and Alzheimer's. Modern Western diets almost certainly do not provide enough of the polyunsaturated omega-3 fats. Aim to include fish in your diet at least twice a week, for example, a main meal of fresh fish not cooked in saturated fat, plus at least one sandwich-sized serving of, say, canned salmon.

Which fish is best?

Oily fish, which tend to have darker-colored flesh and a stronger flavor, are the richest source of omega-3 fats.

Canned fish such as salmon, sardines, mackerel and, to a lesser extent, tuna are all rich sources of omega-3s; look for canned fish packed in water, canola oil, olive oil, tomato sauce, and drain well. The following canned fish contain approximately 650 milligrams of omega-3 fats (considered an adequate daily intake for an adult).

- 1 ounce canned sardines
- 1 ounce canned mackerel
- 1 ounce canned red salmon
- 2 ounces canned pink salmon
- 6 ounces canned tuna

Fresh fish with higher levels of omega-3s are: Atlantic salmon and smoked salmon; Atlantic, Pacific, and Spanish mackerel; southern blue-fin tuna; and swordfish. Eastern and Pacific oysters and squid (calamari) are also rich sources.

Mercury in fish

DUE TO the risk of high levels of mercury in certain species of fish, the Food and Drug Administration (FDA) advises pregnant women, nursing mothers, women planning a pregnancy, and young children to limit fish consumption in their diet to 12 ounces of cooked fish per week, with a typical serving size being

3 to 6 ounces. The species of fish to avoid are shark, swordfish, king mackerel, and tilefish. These long-lived, larger fish contain the highest levels of mercury. Pregnant women should select a variety of other kinds of fish—shellfish, canned fish such as light tuna, or smaller, ocean fish.

5. EAT LESS SATURATED FAT AND REPLACE BAD FATS WITH GOOD FATS

It's not just the quantity of fat in your diet you have to think about—the type of fat can make a big difference to your health, and your waistline. Focus on including the good fats in your diet and minimize foods high in saturated fat and trans-fatty acids.

Our bodies need a certain amount of "good" or unsaturated fat—from nuts, seeds, olives, and avocados, for example—to function properly and thrive. Other fats, called essential fatty acids, can't be manufactured by your body so need to be consumed through your diet. The best sources of these healthy fats are seafood, polyunsaturated oils, mustard seed oil, canola oil, and linseeds.

Replacing saturated fats with monounsaturated and polyunsaturated fats will lower your "bad" cholesterol and increase your "good" cholesterol.

Get rid of bad fats
Minimize saturated fats and oils, including:

- fatty meats and meat products—e.g., sausages, salami
- full-fat dairy products—butter, milk, cream, cheese, ice cream, yogurt

- ghee, coconut, and palm oils
- potato chips, packaged snacks
- cakes, cookies, pastries, pies, pizza
- deep-fried foods—fried chicken, French fries, spring rolls

Choose the good fats

Emphasize the following mono- and polyunsaturated fats in your diet:

- olive, canola, and mustard seed oils
- margarines and spreads made with canola, sunflower, or other seed oils
- avocados
- fish, shellfish, shrimp, scallops, etc.
- walnuts, almonds, cashews, etc.
- olives
- muesli (not toasted)
- flaxseeds

When shopping, look for products low in saturated fat, rather than just low-fat products. The saturated fat content should be less than 20 percent of the total fat.

■

Saturated fat is the main cause of high cholesterol levels. Focus on monounsaturated and omega-3 fats for long-term health.

■

6. MINIMIZE YOUR USE OF SALT

An estimated 75 percent of the salt we eat is not from that which we voluntarily add, but from salt already existing in foods. Bread and butter/margarine, for example, contribute much of the salt we eat. Low-sodium breads take some time to adjust your tastebuds to, but low salt margarines are easy to find on the supermarket shelves and are not noticeably different in taste. Foods high in salt include:

- canned, bottled and packaged soups, sauces, and gravy bases, stock cubes
- sausages, ham, bacon, and other cured meats
- pizza, meat pies, sausage rolls, fried chicken, and other takeout foods
- pickles, chutneys, olives
- snack foods such as potato chips

What does "low-sodium" really mean?

SOME FOODS labeled "low-sodium" are not necessarily low in salt. Always read the label to make sure. According to the FDA, low-salt and low-sodium foods are defined as those with less than 140 mg of sodium per 100 g (or 100 ml for liquids). Look at the nutrition information panel on the package and read the sodium content in the "per 100 g" or "per 100 ml" column. If the sodium content is given in grams instead of milligrams, convert it by multiplying by 1,000 (for example, 1.2 g per 100g = 1200 mg per 100 g).

7. MODERATE YOUR ALCOHOL INTAKE

Of everything we drink, alcohol could be considered the most fattening, not simply because of its calorie content but because it has priority as a fuel over other nutrients. So basically, as long as there's alcohol in your system, anything else is surplus until the alcohol is burned up—and surplus calories are stored, largely as body fat. Looking at it another way, just one can of beer replaces all the calories burnt by 20 minutes of brisk walking.

There is no doubt that large quantities of alcohol should be avoided, but several studies have suggested that a moderate alcohol intake can exert a protective effect against heart disease in some people.

People who drink one or two standard drinks per day, but not necessarily every day, show a reduced risk of heart disease, with the effect being greatest among those with other risk factors for heart disease. It is important to note the finding that three or more drinks per day actually increases the risk of death!

Taking control

THE DIETARY Guidelines for Americans 2005 states those who choose to drink alcoholic beverages should do so sensibly and in moderation—defined as the consumption of up to one drink per day for women and up to two drinks per day for men.

A standard drink is 5 ounces of wine, 12 ounces of beer, 1½ ounces of distilled spirits, and 2 ounces fortified wine such as sherry. For information, counseling or other assistance to help moderate your alcohol intake, contact the drug and alcohol service in your area.

National Institute on Alcohol Abuse and
  Alcoholism
National Institutes of Health
www.niaaa.nih.gov
The National Alcohol and Substance Abuse
  Information Center
www.addictioncareoptions.com
1-800-784-6776

8. INCLUDE NUTS IN YOUR DIET

People who eat nuts once a week have lower levels of heart disease than those who don't eat any nuts. There are probably several reasons for this. Nuts contain: a variety of antioxidants, which keep blood vessels healthy; arginine, an amino acid that helps keep blood flowing smoothly; and folate and fiber, both of which can lower cholesterol levels. Although nuts are high in fat (averaging around 50 percent), it is largely unsaturated, so they make a healthy substitute for foods such as cookies, cakes, pastries, potato chips, and chocolate. Because they are so nutrient and energy dense, a little goes a long way—we suggest you have about 1 ounce most days. They also contain relatively little carbohydrate, so most do not have a GI value.

Some easy ways to eat more nuts
▶ Use nuts in food preparation. For example, use toasted cashews or sesame seeds in a chicken stir-fry, sprinkle walnuts or pine nuts over a salad; top fruity desserts or granola with almonds, add chopped almonds or pecans to muesli.

- Use hazelnut spread on bread or try peanut, almond, or cashew butter rather than butter or margarine.
- Sprinkle a mixture of ground nuts and flaxseeds over cereal or salads, or add to baked goods such as muffins.
- Enjoy a snack of unsalted nuts and dried fruit—just a small handful.

9. USE LOW-FAT DAIRY AND CALCIUM-ENRICHED SOY PRODUCTS

Calcium is the most abundant mineral in our bodies. It builds our bones and teeth and is involved in muscle contraction and relaxation, blood clotting, nerve function, and regulation of blood pressure. If we don't have enough calcium in our diet, our bodies will draw it out of our bones. Over time this can lead to osteoporosis, loss of height, curvature of the spine, and periodontal disease. Research shows that calcium:

- can help lower high blood pressure
- may protect against cancer, particularly cancer of the bladder, bowel, and colon, and possibly against breast, ovarian, pancreas, and skin cancers
- can favorably influence blood fat levels and reduce the risk of stroke
- can reduce the risk of kidney stones
- can assist in weight regulation

Dairy foods are an important source of calcium. They also provide energy, protein, carbohydrate, and vitamins A, B, and D. Virtually all dairy foods have low GI values—largely thanks to lactose, the sugar found naturally in milk, which has a low GI of 46. By choosing low-fat varieties of milk, yogurt, ice cream, and custard, you will enjoy a food that provides you with sustained energy, boosting your calcium intake but not your saturated fat intake. In fact, low-fat milk supplies as much (and usually more) calcium than full-fat milk:

- ◗ 1 cup of low-fat milk contains about 415 mg of calcium and only 0.5 g of fat
- ◗ 1 cup of regular milk contains about 295 mg of calcium and 9.7 g of fat

If you eat only plant foods or want to avoid dairy products, you may turn to soy drinks, yogurts, and desserts. Soy products are not naturally high in calcium, so look for calcium-fortified products if you are relying on them as a source of calcium. Sesame seeds, dried apricots, and figs, Asian greens, and the edible bones of fish also contain calcium.

To meet calcium requirements, experts recommend that adults eat two to three servings of dairy products every day. Good low-fat dairy choices include skim, fat-free or low-fat milk and or low-fat yogurts. A serving is: 1 cup of milk; 1½ ounces of cheese; or 8 ounces of yogurt.

What if you are lactose intolerant?

SOME PEOPLE are lactose intolerant because the enzyme lactase is not active in their small intestine. Children with lactose intolerance often outgrow it by five years of age. If you are lactose intolerant, you should still be able to enjoy cheese—which is virtually lactose free—and yogurt. The microorganisms in yogurt are active in digesting lactose during passage

continued

through the small intestine. Alternatively, try low-lactose, or lactose-free milk and milk products, or low GI, low-fat, calcium-enriched nondairy alternatives such as soy milk. Note that rice milk has a high GI value (92).

10. EAT LEAN RED MEATS AND SKINLESS CHICKEN

▶ Red meat is the best dietary source of iron, the nutrient used in carrying oxygen in our blood, and the main source of zinc, which is a part of over 100 enzymes active in the body. Good iron and zinc status can improve our energy levels and exercise tolerance. A chronic shortage of iron leads to anemia, with symptoms including pale skin, excessive tiredness, breathlessness, and decreased attention span. Even mild iron deficiency can cause unexplained fatigue.

▶ Although chicken contains about one-third the iron of red meat, it is readily absorbed, as it is from red meat, and provides a versatile, nutrient-rich alternative.

▶ Choose lower fat deli meat products such as pastrami, roast beef, low-sodium ham, and rolled turkey breast.

▶ Choose lean cuts of meat.

▶ Cut visible fat from meat and remove skin and underlying fat from poultry before cooking. Drain away the fat after cooking.

What about eggs?

EGGS ALSO contain valuable amounts of the nutrients found in meat, although the iron is not as well absorbed. The cholesterol content of eggs is only a concern if you have high cholesterol levels and/or your total diet is high in saturated fat.

PUTTING THE GI TO WORK IN YOUR DAY

Low GI foods can form the basis of a healthy, flexible diet whoever you are and wherever you live whether you enjoy a traditional American diet or prefer Asian, Indian, or Mediterranean-style cuisines.

Breakfast basics

Follow these breakfast basics to nourish your body and sustain you through the morning. Choose foods from each group—carbohydrate, protein, and fruit and vegetables.

1. Start with a low GI carb such as whole grain breakfast cereal or grainy whole grain bread or toast.
2. Add some protein such as low-fat milk, calcium-enriched soy milk, low-fat yogurt, eggs, reduced-fat cheese, tofu, lean ham, or bacon.
3. Plus fresh, frozen, or canned fruit, dried fruit, fruit or vegetable juice.

Light and easy, the low GI lunch

Take a break and refuel properly at lunchtime to maintain energy levels and concentration throughout the afternoon— and reduce the temptation to snack on something indulgent later in the day.

1. Start with a low GI carb such as whole grain or sourdough bread, pasta, noodles, sweet corn, or legumes.
2. Add some protein such as fresh or canned salmon or tuna, lean meat, sliced chicken, ricotta cheese, or an egg.
3. Plus vegetables or salad to help fill you up. Round off the meal with fruit.

What's for dinner?

What to make for dinner is the perennial question. Most people know that eating well is important, but it can be hard to get motivated to cook at the end of a long day. You don't have to spend hours preparing—if your cupboards and refrigerator are stocked with the right foods, you should be able to put a meal together in under 30 minutes.

1. Start with a low GI carb. What do you feel like? A grain—rice, barley, or cracked wheat? Pasta, noodles, or bean vermicelli? Or perhaps a high carb vegetable such as sweet corn or sweet potato?
2. Add some protein such as lean meat or chicken, fish or seafood, eggs, and legumes. Protein lowers the glycemic load by replacing some of the carbohydrate. It also helps to satisfy the appetite.
3. Plus plenty of vegetables and salad. Round off the meal with fruit.

■

Choose healthy foods you like eating—put them
together to make balanced, low GI meals.

■

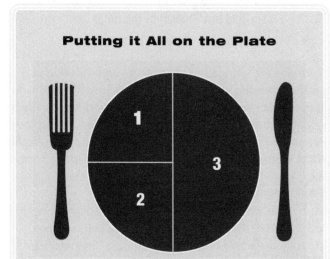

Putting it All on the Plate

1. Carbohydrate
2. Protein
3. Vegetables and salad

The plate model is adaptable to any serving sizes.

As long as the types of food you choose fit within
the "10 Steps to a Healthy Heart Diet" guidelines listed on page 64 then you should have a healthy diet
overall.

A WEEK OF HEART-HEALTHY LOW GI EATING

■

The message for heart disease prevention is low-fat (low saturated fat), high carbohydrate, high fiber, and low GI most of the time!

■

The following week of menus shows you how to achieve a healthy heart diet with a low GI. You can use the menus for ideas for your own meal choices or follow them closely to try out the low GI diet. We have included a couple of between-meal snacks in most of the menus, as they can be part of a normal healthy diet. Each menu is designed to be:

▶ *Low in fat, especially saturated fat*
  We've kept the total amount of fat down to provide less than 30 percent of total calories, according to current recommendations. Saturated fat content is less than 20 grams per day.

▶ *Low in calories*
  These menus provide a total daily energy intake of between 1400 and 1700 calories, which is a minimum amount for most people. Be guided by your appetite to adjust quantities to suit yourself.

▶ *High in carbohydrate with a low GI*
  The carbohydrate content of these menus provides at least 50 percent of total calorie intake. This means an intake of at least 200 grams of carbohydrate each day. The emphasis is on low GI carbohydrate choices.

Generally beverages are included only where they make a significant nutrient or calorie contribution. Supplement the menus with a range of fluids such as water, tea, coffee, herbal tea, mineral water, and soda water with lemon or lime slices.

The quantities in the recipe ideas are a rough guide and can be adjusted to taste.

Allow yourself a treat, occasionally

ALLOW YOURSELF to indulge in a little of whatever takes your fancy occasionally, but only if it is what you really feel like. Indulgences are meant to be enjoyed.

- your favorite cheese and crackers
- a hot dog at the football game
- lean bacon and omega-3 eggs for Sunday brunch
- a takeout meal on Friday night

MONDAY

Total Energy:	1600 Cal
Saturated Fat:	10 g
Carbohydrate:	200 g
Fiber:	45 g

Breakfast: A bowl of All-Bran with a sliced banana and low-fat milk. A slice of grainy toast with unsaturated margarine.

Morning snack: A couple of oatmeal cookies.

Lunch: Two slices of grainy bread filled with tuna, lettuce, and mayonnaise. Follow with a serving of fresh or canned fruit.

Dinner: A large bowl of steaming, thick Minestrone Soup served with crusty Italian bread and a salad with vinaigrette dressing.

Night snack: A small handful of dried fruit and nuts.

Minestrone Soup

Sauté 1 finely chopped onion, 1 thinly sliced leek, and 2 cloves of chopped garlic in a little olive oil. Add 2 diced carrots, 2 sticks of thinly sliced celery, a 14-ounce can of tomatoes, and 1 bay leaf. Add 6 cups of chicken or beef stock, bring to a boil then cover and simmer for 30 minutes. Add a 14-ounce can of cannellini or white beans, ½ cup orzo and simmer for 10–15 minutes. Then add 1 cup fresh or frozen peas and 1 cup shredded cabbage, season with freshly ground black pepper, stir, and cook for a few minutes to heat through.

SERVES 4

TUESDAY

Total Energy:	1600 Cal
Saturated Fat:	10 g
Carbohydrate:	220 g
Fiber:	26 g

Breakfast:	Top a couple of slices of raisin toast with low-fat ricotta cheese and a finely sliced pear. Finish with a skim milk latte.
Lunch:	Black bean tortilla and a cup of fresh pineapple chunks.
Afternoon snack:	A mixed nut bar.
Dinner:	Barbecued Beef Kebabs with basmati rice and a side salad or plenty of steamed vegetables.
Night snack:	Lemon sorbet.

Barbecued Beef Kebabs

Marinate approximately 1 pound diced beef (e.g., rump, fillet) in ½ cup red wine, 1 tablespoon vinegar, 1 tablespoon olive oil, 1 teaspoon Worcestershire sauce, 2 teaspoons tomato sauce, 2 crushed garlic cloves, and black pepper to taste. Thread onto skewers alternately with button mushrooms, diced pepper, and diced onion, and grill or barbecue.

SERVES 4

WEDNESDAY

Total Energy:	1550 Cal
Saturated Fat:	10 g
Carbohydrate:	210 g
Fiber:	25 g

Breakfast:	A bowl of oatmeal with a tablespoon of raisins and low-fat milk. Serve with a glass of orange juice.
Lunch:	Two slices of grainy bread spread with avocado, topped with grated beets, grated carrot, and lettuce. Follow with a piece of fresh fruit and water.
Afternoon snack:	A tub of low-fat yogurt.
Dinner:	Quick Vegetarian Pizza and a side salad.
Night snack:	A small handful (1 ounce) of almonds and a glass of sparkling apple juice.

Quick Vegetarian Pizza

Sauté a diced onion, a clove of crushed garlic, and bell pepper cut into thin strips. Add 4 thinly sliced mushrooms, basil and oregano to taste, and cook for 5 minutes. Stir in a small can ($\frac{1}{2}$ cup) of red kidney beans. Sprinkle a pizza base with $3\frac{1}{2}$ ounces grated reduced-fat mozzarella or cheddar cheese. Spoon the bean mixture over. Pour over about $3\frac{1}{2}$ ounces of bottled tomato purée and top with a further $3\frac{1}{2}$ ounces of cheese. Bake for 10–15 minutes in a hot oven.

SERVES 4

THURSDAY

Total Energy:	1550 Cal
Saturated Fat:	12 g
Carbohydrate:	165 g
Fiber:	33 g

Breakfast:	Toast 2 slices of grainy bread and top with a smear of avocado, sliced tomato, and black pepper. Add a piece of fresh fruit and a drink.
Morning snack:	1 ounce almonds.
Lunch:	Try a bowl of lentil and vegetable soup with flatbread, or pita bread.
Afternoon snack:	An orange.
Dinner:	Salmon Cakes served with a medley of baby corn, snowpeas, sliced carrots, and spring onions. Drizzle with sweet chili sauce, if desired.
Night snack:	Low-fat ice cream in a cone.

Salmon Cakes

Combine 14 ounces canned salmon with half a finely diced onion, 1 cup mashed potato, 2 tablespoons chopped parsley, and 1 large egg. Shape into patties and fry until golden brown on both sides in a pan sprayed with cooking spray.

SERVES 2

FRIDAY

Total Energy:	1500 Cal
Saturated Fat:	10 g
Carbohydrate:	200 g
Fiber:	30 g

Breakfast:	Top a couple of slices of grainy toast with a poached egg. Add a small glass of grapefruit juice or a fresh grapefruit.
Lunch:	Two slices of sourdough rye bread, smear of light cream cheese, sliced smoked salmon, and a side salad.
Afternoon snack:	A slice of raisin toast with a scrape of margarine.
Dinner:	Easy Creamy Pasta with tomato topping and a side salad.
Night snack:	2 thick slices of fresh pineapple.

Easy Creamy Pasta

Cook 14 ounces broad fettuccine in boiling water until al dente. Meanwhile, combine ¼ cup fresh ricotta, ¼ cup low-fat natural yogurt, ¼ cup grated Parmesan cheese, and 3 teaspoons margarine. Stir this mixture through the drained fettuccine, adding some sautéed onion and garlic for extra flavor, if desired.

SERVES 4

SATURDAY

Total Energy:	1570 Cal
Saturated Fat:	10 g
Carbohydrate:	200 g
Fiber:	30 g

Breakfast:	A bowl of Special K with low-fat milk, low-fat berry yogurt, and a handful of strawberries.
Lunch:	A pita bread filled with falafel, hummus, tomato, lettuce, tabbouleh, and chili sauce.
Afternoon snack:	Small bunch of grapes.
Dinner:	Moroccan Lamb and Spicy Rice with plenty of steamed vegetables.
Night snack:	2 fresh plums or an apple.

Moroccan Lamb and Spicy Rice

Cook 1 cup of basmati rice then add 1 cup cooked baby peas. Drain and set aside. Coat about ½ pound lean lamb (e.g., lamb fillet) with a commercial Moroccan spice blend and gently pan-fry in a little olive oil. Remove to a plate and keep warm. In the same pan, sauté a finely sliced onion until golden and soft (don't let it brown), stirring in the spice remaining in the pan. Add the cooked rice and peas, stir to combine and heat through. Serve topped with the lamb cut into strips, with freshly steamed vegetables alongside.

SERVES 4

SUNDAY

Total Energy:	1600 Cal
Saturated Fat:	12 g
Carbohydrate:	160g
Fiber:	30 g

Breakfast:	A bowl of fresh fruit salad topped with 4 ounces low-fat fruit yogurt and a toasted fruit muffin with a scrape of margarine.
Lunch:	An Easy Omelet served with a couple of slices of grainy bread.
Afternoon snack:	A banana.
Dinner:	Pan-fry or barbecue a fish cutlet drizzled with a little olive oil, lemon juice, salt, and pepper. Serve with fresh or canned baby new potatoes and plenty of steamed seasonal vegetables.
Night snack:	A glass of fruit juice and a small scoop of walnuts.

Easy Omelet

Combine 1 whole egg with 2 beaten egg whites. Cook lightly in an omelet pan and top with diced tomato, scallions, and a sprinkle of grated reduced-fat cheese. Finish under the grill.

SERVES 1

More heart-healthy low GI meals

For breakfast

✓ Spread toasted fruit bread with ricotta and top with sliced apple and chopped walnuts.

✓ Enjoy a low-fat berry or mango smoothie.

✓ Spoon fresh peach slices and berries through a tub of low-fat yogurt.

✓ Smear avocado on sourdough and top with tomato slices.

✓ Enjoy a steaming hot chocolate (made with low-fat milk) with whole grain toast and fruit spread.

Lunches that really refuel

✓ Fill some flatbread with hummus and tabbouleh.

✓ Top a tub of fruit salad with a dollop of low-fat yogurt.

✓ Take a green salad plus some bean salad, and add grainy bread.

✓ Sip a cup of steaming homemade minestrone and a piece of fruit.

✓ Tuck into a lentil or veggie burger with chili sauce and salad on a crusty whole grain roll.

✓ Fill a baked potato with baked beans and top with a sprinkle of cheese.

What's for dinner?

✓ Wrap a fish fillet dressed with herbs and lemon, or tomato and onion, in foil and bake. Serve with a heavy grain roll and mixed vegetables or a salad.

✓ Stir-fry lean chicken, meat, or fish with mixed green vegetables. Serve with low GI rice or noodles.

✓ Make a spicy lentil dal and serve with low GI rice and a dollop of chutney.

✓ Top spinach and ricotta tortellini with a tomato sauce and serve with a salad or steamed vegetables.

✓ Create a one-pot chicken casserole with chopped onions, carrots, celery, mushrooms, and potato or sweet potato.

✓ Serve chili beans and beef with soft tortilla bread.

Simple salad combos to serve on the side with a vinaigrette dressing

✓ Mixed garden greens

✓ Carrot with chives or coriander

✓ Cannellini, kidney, and white beans with basil

✓ Tomato, mint, and cucumber

✓ Green beans, arugula, cherry tomatoes, and olives

✓ Radicchio, endive, pears, and walnuts

✓ Chopped celery, apple, and walnuts

✓ Coleslaw with chopped cabbage, grated apples, and carrots

✓ Tabbouleh-bulgur with chopped parsley, mint, tomato and onion

✓ Lentil salad—toss a can of drained lentils and a finely sliced onion in a tangy olive oil and lemon dressing

✓ Celery, walnuts, and lemon thyme

Dessert: a low GI finish

Desserts can make a valuable contribution to your daily calcium and vitamin C intake when they are based on low-fat dairy foods and fruits. If you haven't time to prepare a dessert, why not simply serve a bowl of fruits in season, or a fruit platter with ricotta cheese?

✓ Quick and easy fruit and dairy combos include: low-fat ice cream and strawberries; fresh or canned fruit with low-fat yogurt; sliced banana with low-fat custard; canned blood plums with a dollop of natural yogurt and a sprinkle of toasted muesli

✓ Baked whole apple stuffed with dried fruit

✓ Fruit crisp—top cooked fruit with a crumbled mixture of toasted muesli, wheat flakes, a little melted margarine (mono- or polyunsaturated), and honey

✓ Wrap cooked apple, raisins, currants and a sprinkle of cinnamon in a sheet of filo pastry (brushed with milk, not fat) and bake as a strudel

✓ Make a winter fruit salad with segments of citrus fruits plus raisins soaked in orange juice, honey, and brandy

Sustaining snacks

✓ an apple

✓ an apple and oatbran muffin

✓ dried apricots

✓ a small bowl of cherries or strawberries

✓ low-fat ice cream in a cone

✓ milk, milkshake, or smoothie (low-fat, of course)

✓ 2 to 3 small oatmeal cookies

✓ an orange

✓ ¾ cup orange juice, freshly squeezed

✓ pita bread and a mini-can of bean spread

✓ 1–2 slices raisin toast—try the grain-based fruit loaves

✓ grain bread sandwich with your favorite filling

✓ a bowl of Special K with low-fat milk

✓ a small box of raisins

✓ 8 ounces of low-fat yogurt

MEDITERRANEAN-STYLE DIETS

In the 1980s, scientists were surprised to learn that the rates of heart disease and cancer in parts of Greece, where the traditional diet consisted primarily of fish, fruit, vegetables, olives, and olive oil, were low compared with rates elsewhere in Europe, North America, and other parts of the world. Research since then has shown that Mediterranean-style diets—in countries such as Greece, Italy, southern France, Spain, North Africa, and parts of the Middle East—can lower cholesterol and blood pressure and, therefore, the risk of heart disease. Experts believe the Mediterranean diet is healthy not only because it is lower in saturated fat and higher in monounsaturated fats (found in olives, olive oil, avocados, almonds, pistachios, canola oil, and other foods), but also because it is rich in micronutrients such as folate found in leafy green vegetables.

With its abundance of low GI carbs such as pasta, bulgur, semolina, beans, chickpeas, lentils, and fruit, plus vegetables, nuts, seeds, and seafoods, a Mediterranean diet fits seamlessly into our low GI healthy-heart plan. In addition, meals are often eaten accompanied by a salad with vinaigrette dressing, the acidity of which helps lower the glycemic impact of a meal. The potentially high GI of white bread is reduced by the fact that it is often eaten with low GI foods or dipped in olive oil. As long as total fat intake isn't too high (no more than 30 to 35 percent of total energy), everyone, including people with diabetes, is likely to benefit from a Mediterranean-style diet.

MEDITERRANEAN-STYLE MENU

Breakfast:	Toasted semolina or sourdough bread with baked ricotta, reduced-fat feta or mozzarella cheese, a piece of seasonal fruit, and a low-fat latte
Lunch:	Pasta (cooked until al dente) with pesto sauce and sun-dried tomatoes, a large cucumber, green bean and tomato salad with vinaigrette dressing, plus a glass of sparkling water
Afternoon snack:	Fresh fruit salad
Dinner:	Couscous with Chickpeas, grilled lemon sole (or other white fish filet), and steamed asparagus drizzled with a little balsamic vinegar, plus a small glass of red wine if you wish
Night snack:	A small apple compote topped with chopped walnuts

Couscous with Chickpeas

Place 1 cup medium-grain couscous in a bowl. Add 7 ounces warm water (with a pinch of salt if desired), stirring to make sure it is evenly absorbed. Set aside for about 10 minutes to allow the grains to soften and "plump up." Using a fork or your fingers, gently mix in a tablespoon of olive or canola oil to air the grains and break up any lumps. Stir in a cup of cooked (or canned) chickpeas and heat through over a low heat.

SERVES 2

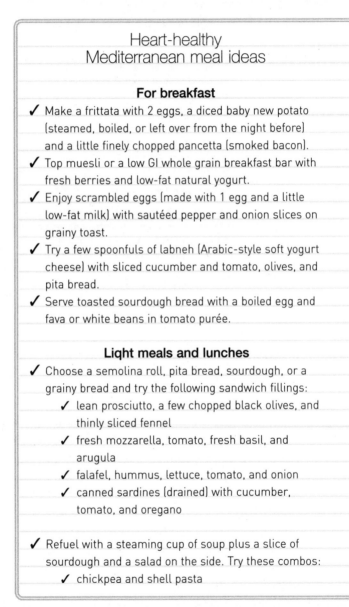

Heart-healthy
Mediterranean meal ideas

For breakfast

✓ Make a frittata with 2 eggs, a diced baby new potato (steamed, boiled, or left over from the night before) and a little finely chopped pancetta (smoked bacon).

✓ Top muesli or a low GI whole grain breakfast bar with fresh berries and low-fat natural yogurt.

✓ Enjoy scrambled eggs (made with 1 egg and a little low-fat milk) with sautéed pepper and onion slices on grainy toast.

✓ Try a few spoonfuls of labneh (Arabic-style soft yogurt cheese) with sliced cucumber and tomato, olives, and pita bread.

✓ Serve toasted sourdough bread with a boiled egg and fava or white beans in tomato purée.

Light meals and lunches

✓ Choose a semolina roll, pita bread, sourdough, or a grainy bread and try the following sandwich fillings:
   - ✓ lean prosciutto, a few chopped black olives, and thinly sliced fennel
   - ✓ fresh mozzarella, tomato, fresh basil, and arugula
   - ✓ falafel, hummus, lettuce, tomato, and onion
   - ✓ canned sardines (drained) with cucumber, tomato, and oregano

✓ Refuel with a steaming cup of soup plus a slice of sourdough and a salad on the side. Try these combos:
   - ✓ chickpea and shell pasta

✓ thick minestrone with elbow pasta

✓ spinach and haricot bean

✓ Make an easy mushroom and parsley omelet with 1 egg and an extra egg white. Serve with a slice of grainy bread and a cannellini bean and red onion salad.

✓ Stuff a large tomato with tuna, diced celery, onion, and low-fat mayonnaise and serve with a bulgur or rice salad topped with toasted pine nuts.

✓ Combine red lentils, low GI rice, chopped onion, garlic, and tomatoes to make a pilaf that's delicious hot or cold.

✓ Enjoy a Turkish pizza pita (Turkish flatbread) filled with meat and lots of chopped tomato, onion, and pepper.

What's for dinner?

✓ Serve al dente angel hair with seafood mix (mussels, clams, squid, shrimp) tossed in a pan with garlic, parsley, chili, and olive oil. Team with a green salad.

✓ Toss al dente penne pasta with seared chunks of fresh tuna and a sauce of black olives, capers, minced fresh herbs, and olive oil. Serve a salad on the side.

✓ Layer baked or grilled eggplant slices, low-fat mozzarella cheese, and tomato purée in a baking dish then sprinkle with a little Parmesan cheese and bake until the mozzarella has melted. Serve with toasted crostini (thinly sliced toasted semolina or sourdough bread) spread with olive oil, pesto or olive tapenade, plus a tossed salad.

✓ Roast chicken with rosemary and serve with ribbon pasta (tagliatelle, fettuccine) tossed in pesto sauce and topped with sun-dried tomatoes and some steamed broccoli on the side.

✓ Lightly sauté a veal scaloppine and serve with orzo (rice-shaped) pasta and pinto beans, tomatoes, and onions and lightly steamed cauliflower.

✓ Serve spaghetti with fresh tomato and basil sauce, beef and ricotta meatballs, plus sautéed zucchini and onion slices with fresh mint.

✓ Roast a leg of lamb and serve with steamed basmati rice and a vegetable stew made with tomatoes, bell peppers, and onions.

✓ Enjoy a veal stew with peas, carrots, and artichoke hearts served with lightly pan-fried baby new potato slices in rosemary and garlic alongside a tossed green salad.

✓ Try chicken tagine with couscous, spinach dressed in lemon and olive oil, and a mixed green salad with vinaigrette.

✓ Combine lamb kofta (spicy meatballs) with minted yogurt, rice pilaf, and tabbouleh.

✓ Grill calamari with fresh lemon juice and serve with white beans in a fresh tomato salsa, plus steamed green vegetables.

✓ Stuff cabbage leaves with rice, tomato, onion, and bell pepper, and serve with natural yogurt and a tomato, black olive, and onion salad.

✓ Make a lamb, carrot, and green casserole and serve with baked orzo pasta in a tomato purée, and a mixed leaf and onion salad on the side.

Desserts: a low GI finish

✓ Stewed peach halves stuffed with crushed amaretti (almond paste macaroons) and a little melted margarine.

- ✓ A fresh fruit crepe with apple, pear, plum, and nectarine, sprinkled with a little sugar.
- ✓ Fresh fruit salad macerated in red or white wine and nutmeg.
- ✓ Stewed pears with a drizzle of chocolate sauce.
- ✓ A scoop of ice cream with cherry compote.
- ✓ Fresh berries with a scoop of ice cream.
- ✓ Strawberries macerated in balsamic vinegar.
- ✓ Fresh fruit salad of cantaloupe, watermelon, strawberries, and pineapple.
- ✓ Thick natural yogurt drizzled with honey and served with grilled peaches.
- ✓ Grilled figs with cinnamon and ice cream.
- ✓ Baked custard topped with filo pastry and honey syrup.
- ✓ Poached peaches or pears in white wine and nutmeg.

Sustaining snacks

- ✓ Grapes and toasted almonds.
- ✓ Pita bread pizzetta ("little pizza": tomato paste, reduced-fat mozzarella, oregano).
- ✓ Semolina or sourdough crostini with olive, artichoke, or red pepper tapenade.
- ✓ Cherries and mixed berries with vanilla or lemon low-fat yogurt.
- ✓ A handful of dried apricots, dates, and figs.
- ✓ A small bowl of sunflower and pumpkin seeds.
- ✓ Thick natural low-fat yogurt drizzled with honey.
- ✓ A handful of mixed unsalted nuts.
- ✓ Babaganoush (eggplant dip) and tzatziki (cucumber dip) served with toasted pita bread triangles.

ASIAN-STYLE DIETS

People living a traditional, rural way of life throughout Asia have low rates of heart disease and type 2 diabetes, and are less likely than those people living in urbanized, Western countries to become overweight or obese as they age. Why? It could be because they eat a high carbohydrate, plant-based diet and get lots of physical activity. Asian-style diets contain a good deal of rice; in fact, people in Asian countries consume rice—usually white—in large amounts at all meals. This eating style fits in perfectly with our low GI heart-healthy plans, since along with the rice, people in much of Asia also eat small amounts of some lean meat, poultry, or fish, in addition to vegetables and fruit.

In India, one low-fat, low GI food—dal—often accompanies meals. Many Asian diets are low in fat and relatively rich in omega-3 fats. Japanese people, for example, regularly eat fish and seaweed, both good sources of these essential fatty acids.

There are other benefits to Asian-style diets, too. Because meat and fish are expensive, Asian people usually include lots of soybeans, other vegetables, and sometimes seaweed with their rice. From a health perspective, these additional vegetables may be the most important component of the Asian diet, since vegetables are full of micronutrients, vitamins, minerals, and phytochemicals.

Asian-style diets differ from Western diets in many ways, one of which is the abovementioned proportion of plant to animal foods. In the following menu, the protein content comes more from plants than from animal sources, and the rice and noodles keep the carbohydrate content high.

■

Soybeans have one of the lowest GI values of any food. When you add them to meals and snacks, you reduce the overall GI of your diet and gain important health benefits.

■

RICE

CARB-RICH rice is one of the oldest and most cultivated grains—there are some 2,000 varieties worldwide—and the staple food for over half the world's population. A soup, salad, or stir-fry based around rice with a little fish, chicken, tofu, or lean meat and plenty of vegetables will give you a healthy balance of carbs, fat, and protein plus some fiber and essential vitamins and minerals. As with pasta and noodles, it's easy to eat too much rice, so keep portions moderate. Even when you choose a low GI rice, eating too much can have a marked effect on your blood glucose levels. A cup of cooked rice combined with plenty of mixed vegetables can turn into three cups of a rice-based meal that suits any adult's daily diet.

Rice can have a very high GI value, or a low one, depending on the variety and its amylose content. Amylose is a kind of starch that resists gelatinization. Although rice is a whole grain food, when you cook it the millions of microscopic cracks in the grains let water penetrate right to the middle of the grain, allowing the starch granules to swell and become fully gelatinized, thus very easy to digest.

continued

So, if you are a big rice eater, opt for the low GI varieties with a higher amylose content, such as basmati or Uncle Ben's converted long-grain rice. These high-amylose rices that stay firm and separate when cooked combine well with Indian, Thai, and Vietnamese cuisines.

Arborio risotto rice releases its starch during cooking and has a medium GI. Brown rice is an extremely nutritious form of rice and contains several B vitamins, minerals, dietary fiber, and protein. Chewier than regular white rice, it tends to take about twice as long to cook. The varieties that have been tested to date have a high GI, so enjoy it occasionally, especially combined with low GI foods such as legumes.

Sushi rice (GI 48) is a short-grain rice with a slightly sticky, soft texture when cooked. Wild rice (GI 57) is not actually rice at all, but a type of grass seed.

ASIAN-STYLE MENU

Breakfast:	Tofu and spinach soup with noodles
Morning snack:	Large apple or pear
Lunch:	Stir-fried Chinese broccoli with beef strips and steamed rice
Afternoon snack:	Soy drink and fresh fruit
Dinner:	Ginger-seasoned fish with carrots, bamboo shoots, celery, and glazed green beans, plus steamed rice and seasonal fruit salad
Night snack:	Handful of almonds

Heart health and eating out Asian-style

When eating out in Asian restaurants, opt for:

- steamed dumplings, dim sum, or fresh spring rolls rather than fried entrées
- clear soups to fill you up, rather than high fat laksas
- noodles in soups rather than fried in dishes such as pad Thai
- noodle and vegetable stir-fries—if you ask for extra vegetables you may find that the one dish feeds two!
- seafood braised in a sauce with plenty of vegetables
- tofu (bean curd), chicken, beef, lamb, or pork fillet braised with nuts and vegetables
- salads such as tangy Thai and Vietnamese salads
- smaller servings of rice
- vegetable dishes such as stir-fried vegetables, vegetable curry, dal, channa (a chickpea curry), and side orders such as pickles, cucumber and yogurt, tomato, and onion
- Japanese dishes such as sushi, teriyaki, sashimi, and pan-seared salmon or tuna; or teppanyaki, which is cooked on a grill, in preference to deep-fried tempura

Heart-healthy Asian-style meal ideas

For breakfast

Chinese

✓ Combine a small serving of steamed low GI rice with soy, egg, and plenty of steamed water spinach.

✓ Stir fresh rice noodles into a bowl of a clear chicken soup with shredded cooked chicken (skin removed), shallots, minced ginger, and winter melon.

✓ Dry-fry a little leftover low GI rice with a fresh diced tomato and a beaten egg, drizzle with light soy sauce, and top with generous snippets of garlic chives (about a quarter of a bunch).

✓ Top steamed egg and minced pork custard with lots of steamed Chinese spinach. Add a small bowl of steamed low GI rice.

Southeast Asian

✓ Make congee (rice porridge) with shredded chicken, pork, shrimp, or fish, stock, chopped shallots, ginger, coriander, garlic, and fish sauce.

✓ Enjoy laska (spicy soup) made with chicken, fish, or pork and mung bean vermicelli noodles—use a table-spoon of light coconut milk per serving.

✓ Server scrambled eggs with a crusty bread roll.

Indian

✓ Try semolina *umpa* topped with lentils that have been soaked then quickly dry-cooked and chopped nuts. Serve with a bowl of low-fat natural yogurt.

✓ Sprinkle spicy whole green gram with finely chopped green chili, lime juice, and chopped onions.

✓ Top namkeen chila pancakes made from besan (chickpea) flour with chopped onions, tomatoes, and coriander leaves and serve them hot with minty chutney, tomato sauce, and low-fat natural yogurt.

Light meals and lunches

Chinese

✓ Steam skinless chicken and tatsoi and serve with a little low GI rice plus clear chicken soup with minced ginger, garlic, and chili, plus shallots and sesame oil on the side.

✓ Dry-fry rice noodles with shredded beef, bean sprouts, Chinese broccoli, and dark soy sauce.

✓ Toss mung bean vermicelli with shredded skinless duck, Chinese cabbage, and hoisin sauce.

✓ Serve two-minute noodles (choose low-fat ones) with bok choy, lean red barbequed pork, and shredded bamboo shoots.

✓ Combine steamed low GI rice with preserved fish, bean curd, Chinese mushrooms, and bok choy.

Southeast Asian

✓ Make a Thai beef salad—grilled slices of lean beef served on a bed of mung bean vermicelli, mint leaves, cucumber, and tomato and dressed with lemon juice, fish sauce, and chili.

✓ Fill rice paper rolls with pork strips (marinated in ginger, soy, and a little sesame oil), sliced bell peppers, carrot, coriander, and snow pea sprouts. Serve with a sweet chili dipping sauce.

✓ Make Thai stuffed omelet—minced chicken with onion and tomato wrapped in an omelet (coat the frying pan with spray olive or canola oil)—and serve with a side salad of grated carrot, bell pepper, and cucumber slices.

✓ Enjoy pho (Vietnamese noodle soup) made with strips of lean beef, scallions, ginger, black pepper, bean shoots, mung bean vermicelli, and fish sauce.

✓ Stir-fry low GI noodles with tofu, scrambled egg, onion, bok choy, bean shoots, and soy sauce.

✓ Serve Thai-style fish cakes on a salad of shredded lettuce, grated carrot, cucumber, bean sprouts, and mint leaves dressed in a sweet chili sauce.

Indian

✓ Serve rajmah (kidney bean cooked with chopped garlic, ginger, and onions) over basmati rice, with sabji (cooked vegetables) such as boiled or steamed baby new potatoes and green fenugreek leaves and cucumber, lettuce, and tomato salad on the side.

✓ Thread fish pieces marinated in tandoori paste and button mushrooms alternately on skewers, and grill or barbecue. Serve with basmati rice and low-fat natural yogurt.

✓ Serve whole wheat rotis with dal of red lentils cooked in onions and tomato plus low-fat yogurt and cauliflower florets and diced carrots gently cooked in canola oil.

✓ Bake whole tomatoes stuffed with garam masala-spiced ricotta cheese and serve with low GI rice with cooked lentils and soybeans, plus a cucumber and onion salad.

✓ Serve whole wheat rotis and chopped green fenugreek leaves with cooked tomato, a grilled chicken drumstick (skin removed), low-fat natural yogurt, and a side salad.

What's for dinner?

Chinese

Chinese dinners traditionally consist of several courses—soup, a protein dish (or dishes), a vegetable dish (or dishes), rice, and a fruit plate. If you keep your food choices to the proportions shown on page 84, your meal will be balanced. Try these heart-healthy low GI dinner combinations (all served with a small bowl of steamed low GI rice):

✓ Bitter melon soup with black-eyed beans and dried scallops; stir-fried chicken (small pieces) with asparagus and black beans; stir-fried Chinese broccoli.

✓ Tofu and fresh pea soup; whole snapper steamed with ginger, shallots, coriander, and soy sauce; stir-fried snake beans with garlic and chili.

✓ Fish head soup with water spinach; Mongolian lamb with leeks; steamed Chinese mushrooms and cabbage.

✓ Sweet and sour tofu soup; steamed lean pork ribs with black bean sauce; stir-fried green beans, baby corn, and water chestnuts.

✓ Clear beef and carrot soup; shredded barbecue duck (skinless) salad with cucumber, agar-agar, shallots, and sesame seeds; Chinese cabbage and button mushrooms "creamed style" with chicken stock and dried scallops.

✓ Gai choy (Chinese mustard greens) soup; honey-soy braised soybeans; stir-fried shrimp with broccoli, bamboo shoots, and cloud ear fungus.

Southeast Asian

✓ Grill lean pork chops marinated in fish sauce, sugar, shallots, and garlic. Serve with steamed low GI rice

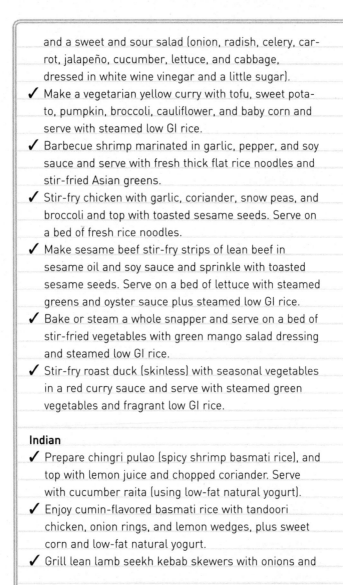

and a sweet and sour salad (onion, radish, celery, carrot, jalapeño, cucumber, lettuce, and cabbage,
dressed in white wine vinegar and a little sugar).

✓ Make a vegetarian yellow curry with tofu, sweet potato, pumpkin, broccoli, cauliflower, and baby corn and
serve with steamed low GI rice.

✓ Barbecue shrimp marinated in garlic, pepper, and soy
sauce and serve with fresh thick flat rice noodles and
stir-fried Asian greens.

✓ Stir-fry chicken with garlic, coriander, snow peas, and
broccoli and top with toasted sesame seeds. Serve on
a bed of fresh rice noodles.

✓ Make sesame beef stir-fry strips of lean beef in
sesame oil and soy sauce and sprinkle with toasted
sesame seeds. Serve on a bed of lettuce with steamed
greens and oyster sauce plus steamed low GI rice.

✓ Bake or steam a whole snapper and serve on a bed of
stir-fried vegetables with green mango salad dressing
and steamed low GI rice.

✓ Stir-fry roast duck (skinless) with seasonal vegetables
in a red curry sauce and serve with steamed green
vegetables and fragrant low GI rice.

Indian

✓ Prepare chingri pulao (spicy shrimp basmati rice), and
top with lemon juice and chopped coriander. Serve
with cucumber raita (using low-fat natural yogurt).

✓ Enjoy cumin-flavored basmati rice with tandoori
chicken, onion rings, and lemon wedges, plus sweet
corn and low-fat natural yogurt.

✓ Grill lean lamb seekh kebab skewers with onions and

button mushrooms and serve with basmati rice and low-fat natural yogurt.

✓ Serve hot bajra (barley) chapatis with palak paneer (spinach cooked with cottage cheese) and low-fat raita, made with cucumber, onion, and nuts.

✓ Combine a plate of steamed idlis (a South Indian dish made from fermented rice and black gram dhal) with hot sambhar dhal made with lentils, chopped steamed peppers, green chili, and curry leaves.

Desserts: a low GI finish

Chinese

Serve a plate of sliced fruit after the main meal. Desserts such as a sweet soup or little delicacies are for special occasions. To reduce the overall GI of sweet treats, try replacing the yellow rock sugar with a low GI pure floral honey, locally grown.

✓ Candied walnuts—dry-roasted walnuts drizzled with pure floral honey and sprinkled with sesame seeds.

✓ Almond soup—freshly ground almonds, rice, and mandarin peel heated with milk and sweetened with honey.

✓ Sweet tofu—make a sweet syrup using apple juice or the unsweetened juice from canned fruit and pour around soft tofu.

✓ Dried tofu sheets, water chestnuts, and egg flower sweet clear soup.

✓ Water chestnut cake.

✓ Red-bean paste cake with a walnut cookie.

Southeast Asian

✓ Low-fat coconut ice cream with sliced banana.

✓ Fruit salad of pineapple, pawpaw, and banana drizzled with passion fruit pulp.

✓ Low-fat lychee ice cream.

✓ Sago pudding—use low-fat milk and be sparing with the sugar.

Indian

✓ A glass of refreshing mango lassi made with low-fat ice cream and skim milk blended with ripe sweet mango and topped with grated almonds.

✓ A plate of saffron-flavored creamy kulfi (traditional ice cream) made with low-fat milk and low-fat sweetened condensed milk, topped with cashews, pistachios, and walnuts. Serve with strawberries.

✓ A banana and some berries blended with low-fat milk (or low-fat vanilla-flavored milk) and a few drops of pure floral honey, and served topped with chopped almonds and walnuts.

✓ Steamed cardamom-flavored semolina pudding made from low-fat milk sweetened with pure floral honey and topped with raisins, pistachios, and almonds.

✓ An apple baked with a drizzle of pure floral honey.

Sustaining snacks

Chinese

✓ A custard apple

✓ A handful of unsalted peanuts

✓ A handful of dried fruit

✓ Mandarin and orange segments

Southeast Asian
✓ Roasted soybeans
✓ Pumpkin seeds
✓ Dried taro
✓ Pomelo grapefruit segments

Indian
✓ Mashed potato and sweet potato patties coated with coriander chutney and topped with chickpea chole, along with low-fat natural yogurt and tomato sauce.
✓ Triangular sandwiches: low GI bread with green coriander chutney on one side and tomato sauce on the other.
✓ A sambhar of lentils and steamed vegetables served on steamed semolina idlis and topped with chopped cashews and walnuts and green chutney.

PART 4

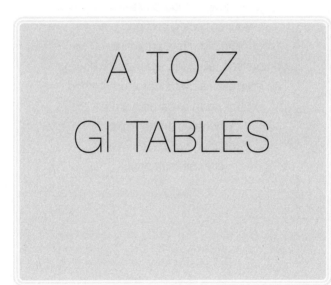

A TO Z
GI TABLES

These A to Z
tables will help you
put low GI food choices into
your shopping cart and onto
your plate. To make an absolutely fair
comparison, all foods are tested following
an internationally standardized method.
Gram for gram of carbohydrates, the
higher the GI, the higher
the blood glucose levels
after consumption.

■

A low GI value is 55 or less
A medium GI value is 56 to 69 inclusive
A high GI value is 70 or more

■

To give you the full picture of the glycemic impact of foods, the tables in this book also include the GL (glycemic load) of average-sized portions of the food on your plate. Glycemic load is the product of the GI and the amount of carbohydrate in a serving of food. If you eat an exceptionally large portion of a low GI food, the GL can be high. This doesn't negate the low GI benefits of the food but it does increase the glycemic impact.

Caution: while low GI is generally associated with healthful diets, low GL may not be. A low GL diet could be full of butter and fatty meat or high in whole grains, fruit, and vegetables. Low GI is a better target than low GL.

Use the GI values in the tables to:
- identify the best carbohydrate choices
- find the GI of your favorite foods
- compare carb-rich foods within a category (two types of bread or breakfast cereal, for example)
- improve your diet by finding a low GI substitute for high GI foods

> ▶ put together a low GI meal
> ▶ help you calculate the GL of a meal or serving if it is more or less than our specified nominal portion size

Use the GL values in the tables to:

> ▶ find foods with a high GI but low carbohydrate content per serving

Remember, the GL values listed in these tables are for the specified nominal portion size. If you eat more (or less) you will need to calculate another GL value.

We have also included some foods that contain very little carbohydrate or none at all because so many people ask us for their GI. Many vegetables such as avocado and broccoli, and protein-rich foods such as eggs, cheese, chicken, and tuna, are among the low or no carbohydrate category. Most alcoholic beverages are also low in carbohydrate.

> ★ indicates that this food contains little or no carbohydrate

In addition, not all low GI foods are a good choice; some are too high in saturated fat and sodium for everyday eating.

> ■ indicates that this food is high in saturated fat

As we have mentioned before, the GI should not be used in isolation—the overall nutritional value of the food needs to be considered.

If you can't find the GI value for a food you regularly eat in these tables, check out our Web site (www.glycemic index.com). We maintain an international database of published GI values that have been tested by a reliable laboratory.

Alternatively, contact the manufacturer and encourage them to have the food tested by an accredited laboratory. In the meantime, choose a similar food from the tables as a substitute.

Look for the GI on the foods you buy

Some foods show a GI value on the label. Unfortunately, not all claims are reliable.

The GI Symbol Program

*

This symbol on foods is your guarantee that the product meets the GI Symbol Program's strict nutritional criteria. Whether high, medium, or low GI, you can be assured that these foods are healthy choices within their food group and will make a nutritious contribution to your diet.

The GI Symbol Program is an international program that was established by the University of Sydney, Diabetes Australia, and the Juvenile Diabetes Research Foundation-organizations whose expertise in GI is recognized around the world. The logo is a trademark of the University of Sydney in Australia and in other countries including the UK. A food product carrying this logo is nutritious and has been tested for its GI in an accredited laboratory. For more information, visit www.gisymbol.com

* ©® and ™ University of Sydney in Australia and other countries.
   All rights reserved.

Note: The GI values in this book are correct at the time of publication. However, the formulation of commercial foods can change, which may lead to a change in the GI of that food.

GI News

To stay up to date with glycemic index research, check out the official glycemic index newsletter, GI News: http://ginews.blogspot.com

Food	GI Glucose = 100	Nominal Serving Size	Available Carbs per Serving	GL per Serving
Alfalfa sprouts, raw	*	½ cup	0	0
All-Bran®, breakfast cereal, Kellogg's®	34	½ cup	15	4
Angel food cake, plain	67■	2 ounces (⅛ cake)	29	19
Apple, dried	29	2 ounces	34	10
Apple, fresh	38	1 small (4 ounces)	15	6
Apple muffin, homemade	46■	1 small (2 ounces)	29	13
Apricot-filled fruit bar, made with whole grain flour	50■	1¾ ounces	34	17
Apricot fruit spread, reduced-sugar	55	1 Tbsp.	6	4
Apricot jam, 100% fruit	50	1 Tbsp.	9	5
Apricots, canned in light syrup	64	½ cup	19	12
Apricots, dried	30	2 ounces	28	9
Apricots, fresh	57	3 small (6 ounces)	13	7
Arborio, risotto rice, white, boiled	69	¾ cup	43	29
Artichokes, globe, fresh or canned	★	½ cup	0	0
Aruglua	★	1 cup	0	0
Asparagus	★	½ cup	0	0
Avocado	★	2 Tbsp.	0	0
Bacon, lean	★	2 medium strips (½ ounce)	0	0
Bagel, white	72	1 small (2½ ounces)	35	25
Baked beans, canned in tomato sauce, Heinz®	55	½ cup	17	8
Banana bread, homemade	51½	1 slice (3 ounces)	38	18
Banana, ripe	52	1 small (4 ounces)	26	13
Banana smoothie, soy drink, low-fat	30	8 fluid ounces	22	7

★ little or no carbs   ■ high in saturated fat

Food	GI Glucose = 100	Nominal Serving Size	Available Carbs per Serving	GL per Serving
Barley, pearled, boiled	25	1 cup	32	8
Basmati rice, white, boiled	58	¾ cup	38	22
Bean sprouts, raw	★	½ cup	0	0
Beef, cooked	★■	3 ounces	0	0
Beer (4.6% alcohol)	66	8 fluid ounces	10	0
Beets, red, canned	64	½ cup	7	5
Bell Peppers	★	½ cup	0	0
Black beans, boiled	30	¾ cup	25	5
Black bean soup, canned	64	1 cup	27	17
Blackberry jam, 100% fruit	46	1 Tbsp.	9	4
Black-eyed peas, boiled	42	¾ cup	29	12
Blueberry muffin, commercially made	59½	1 small (2 ounces)	29	17
Bok choy	★	½ cup	0	0
Bran Flakes™, breakfast cereal, Kellogg's®	74	¾ cup	18	13
Bran muffin, commercially made	60½	1 small (2 ounces)	24	15

BREAD

Food	GI Glucose = 100	Nominal Serving Size	Available Carbs per Serving	GL per Serving
9 Grain, multigrain bread [G]	43	1 slice	14	6
Bagel, white	72	1 small (2½ ounces)	35	25
Country grain and organic rye bread [G]	48	1 slice	10	5
Dinner roll, white	73	1 small (1 ounce)	16	12
Flaxseed and soy bread [G]	36	1 slice	9	3
Gluten-free multigrain bread	79	1 slice	13	10
Hamburger bun, white	61	½ bun (1 ounce)	15	9
Kaiser roll, white	73	½ roll (1 ounce)	16	12
Lebanese bread, white	75	1 ounce	16	12
Melba toast, plain	70	1 ounce	23	16

★ little or no carbs ■ high in saturated fat

Food	GI Glucose = 100	Nominal Serving Size	Available Carbs per Serving	GL per Serving
Multigrain sandwich bread, enriched	65	1 slice	28	18
Oat bran and honey bread [G]	49	1 slice	13	7
Organic stoneground whole wheat sourdough bread	59	1 slice	12	7
Pita bread, 4" white	57	1 ounce	17	10
Pumpernickel bread	50	1 slice	10	5
Raisin bread	63	1 slice	17	11
Rye bread, black	76	1 slice	13	10
Rye bread, light	68	1 slice	14	10
Rye bread, whole grain	58	1 slice	14	8
Sourdough rye bread	48	1 slice	12	6
Sourdough wheat bread	54	1 slice	14	8
Spelt multigrain bread	54	1 slice	12	7
Stuffing, bread	74	½ cup	21	16
Sunflower and barley bread	57	1 slice	11	6
White bread, enriched, sliced	71	1 slice	14	10
Whole wheat bread, made w/enriched wheat flour, sliced	71	1 slice	12	9
Whole wheat bread, 100%, stoneground	59	1 slice	12	7
Wonder White®, bread, sliced	80	1 slice	15	12

BREAKFAST CEREALS

Food	GI Glucose = 100	Nominal Serving Size	Available Carbs per Serving	GL per Serving
All-Bran®, Kellogg's®	34	½ cup	15	5
Bran Flakes, Kellogg's®	74	¾ cup	18	13
Cocoa Krispies®, Kellogg's®	77	1 cup	26	20
Corn Flakes®, Kellogg's®	77	1 cup	25	20
Corn Pops®, Kellogg's®	80	1 cup	26	21
Crispix®	87	1 cup	25	22
Froot Loops®, Kellogg's®	69	1 cup	26	18
Frosted Flakes®, Kellogg's®	55	1 cup	26	15
Gluten-free muesli, with 2% fat milk	39	¼ cup	19	7
Honey Smacks®, Kellogg's®	71	1 cup	23	16
Muesli, natural	40	¼ cup	18	8
Muesli, toasted	43	¼ cup	17	7

★ little or no carbs   ■ high in saturated fat

Food	GI Glucose = 100	Nominal Serving Size	Available Carbs per Serving	GL per Serving
Muesli, Swiss Formula	56	¼ cup	16	9
Nutri-Grain™, Kellogg's®	66	½ cup	15	10
Oat bran, raw, unprocessed	55	2 Tbsp.	5	3
Oatmeal, instant, made with water	82	1 cup	26	17
Oatmeal, from old-fashioned rolled oats, made with water	58	1 cup	21	11
Oatmeal, from steel-cut oats, made with water	52	1 cup	22	11
Puffed buckwheat	65	1 cup	12	8
Puffed rice	80	2 cups	21	17
Puffed wheat	80	2 cups	21	17
Rice bran, unprocessed	19	4 Tbsp.	14	3
Raisin Bran, Kellogg's®	73	½ cup	19	14
Rice Krispies®, Kellogg's®	82	1¼ cups	26	22
Semolina, wheat, hot cereal, made with water	55	⅔ cup	11	6
Shredded Wheat	75	½ cup	20	15
Special K®, regular, Kellogg's®	56	1 cup	21	11
Weetabix®, biscuits, regular	69	½ cup	17	12
Breton wheat crackers	67■	1 ounce	14	10
Fava beans	79	½ cup	11	9
Broccoli	★	½ cup	0	0
Brussels sprouts	★	½ cup	0	0
Buckwheat, groats, boiled	54	¾ cup	30	16
Buckwheat pancakes, 6", gluten-free, from pancake mix	102	1 pancake	22	22
Buckwheat, puffed	65	1 cup	12	8
Bulgur, cracked wheat, ready to eat	48	½ cup	26	12
Bun, hamburger, white	61	½ bun (1 ounce)	15	9
Butter beans, canned	36	¼ cup	12	4
Butter beans, dried, boiled	31	½ cup	20	6
Cabbage	★	½ cup	0	0
Calamari or squid, not battered or breaded	★	3 ounces	0	0
Cannellini beans	31	½ cup	12	4

★ little or no carbs ■ high in saturated fat

Food	GI Glucose = 100	Nominal Serving Size	Available Carbs per Serving	GL per Serving
Cantaloupe	67	½ cup	6	4
Capellini pasta, white, boiled	45	1 cup	45	20
Carrot juice, freshly made	43	8 fluid ounces	23	10
Carrots, peeled, cooked	41	½ cup	5	2
Cashew nuts, salted	22	1 ounce	9	2
Cauliflower	★	½ cup	0	0
Celery	★	½ cup	0	0
Cheese	★■	1 ounce	0	0
Cheese curls, cheese-flavored snack	74■	2 ounces	29	22
Cheese tortellini, cooked	50■	6 ounces	21	10
Cherries, dark, raw	63	1 cup	12	3
Chicken, without the skin and bone	★	4 ounces	0	0
Chicken nuggets, frozen, reheated	46■	3½ ounces	16	7
Chickpeas, canned	40	½ cup	22	9
Chickpeas, dried, boiled	28	¾ cup	24	7
Chilies, fresh or dried	★	2 Tbsp.	0	0
Chives, fresh	★	2 Tbsp.	0	0
Chocolate cake, made from package mix, frosting, Betty Crocker	38■	½ cake (3 ounces)	52	20
Chocolate-coated cookie, gluten-free	35	1 ounce	14	5
Chocolate hazelnut smoothie, low-fat	34	8 fluid ounces	25	8
Chocolate ice cream, low-fat [G]	49	½ cup	14	7
Chocolate pudding, instant, made from package with whole milk	47■	½ cup	16	7
Coca-Cola®, soft drink	53	8 fluid ounces	26	14
Cocoa Krispies®, breakfast cereal, Kellogg's®	77	1 cup	26	20
Condensed milk, sweetened, full-fat	61■	2 ounces	28	17
Consommé, clear, chicken or vegetable	★	1 cup	2	0

★ little or no carbs   ■ high in saturated fat

Food	GI Glucose = 100	Nominal Serving Size	Available Carbs per Serving	GL per Serving
Corn chips, plain, salted	42■	1¾ ounces	25	11
Corn Flakes®, breakfast cereal, Kellogg's®	77	1 cup	25	20
Cornmeal (polenta), boiled	68	⅔ cup	13	9
Corn pasta, gluten-free, boiled, Orgran	78	1¼ cups	42	32
Corn Pops®, breakfast cereal, Kellogg's®	80	1 cup	26	21
Corn, sweet, on the cob, boiled	48	1 medium ear	16	8
Corn, sweet, whole kernel, canned, drained	46	⅓ cup	14	7
Couscous, boiled	65	1 cup	33	21
Cranberries, dried, sweetened	64	1½ ounces	29	19
Cranberry Juice Cocktail, Ocean Spray	52	8 fluid ounces	31	16
Crispix®, breakfast cereal, Kellogg's®	87	1 cup	25	22
Croissant, plain	67■	2 ounces	26	17
Cupcake, strawberry-iced	73■	1 ounce	26	19
Cherimoya, fresh, flesh only	54	1 small (4 ounces)	19	10
Custard, reduced-fat, vanilla	37	½ cup	15	6
Custard, traditional, homemade	43■	½ cup	17	7
Dates, Arabic, dried, vacuum-packed	39	2 ounces	41	16
Dates, fresh	103	2 ounces	40	42
Diet jelly	★	2 Tbsp.	0	0
Diet soft drinks	★	8 fluid ounces	0	0
Digestives® cookies, plain	59	1 ounce	16	10
Dried apple	29	2 ounces	34	10
Duck, without the skin and bone	★■	3 ounces	0	0
Eggplant	★	½ cup	0	0
Eggs	★	2 eggs	0	0
Endive	★	1 cup	0	0
Fanta®, orange soft drink	68	8 fluid ounces	34	23

★ little or no carbs   ■ high in saturated fat

Food	GI Glucose = 100	Nominal Serving Size	Available Carbs per Serving	GL per Serving
Fennel	★	½ cup	0	0
Fettuccine, egg noodle, cooked	40	1 cup	46	18
Figs, dried	61	2 ounces	26	16
Fish, all-types, fresh or frozen, without skin	★	3 ounces	0	0
Fish sticks, lightly breaded	38½	3 ounces	19	7
French fries, frozen, baked	75½	5 ounces	29	22
French vanilla ice cream, full fat	38½	½ cup	9	3
Froot Loops®, breakfast cereal, Kellogg's®	69	1 cup	26	18
Frosted Flakes®, breakfast cereal, Kellogg's®	55	¾ cup	26	15
Fructose, pure	19	1 Tbsp.	10	2
Garlic	★	1 clove	0	0
Gatorade® sports drink	78	8 fluid ounces	15	12
Gelati, sugar-free, chocolate	37	1 cup	14	5
Gelati, sugar-free, vanilla	39	1 cup	14	5
Ginger, grated	★	1 tsp.	0	0
Golden syrup	63	1 Tbsp.	17	11
Granny Smith apple juice, unsweetened	44	8 fluid ounces	24	10
Grapefruit, fresh	25	½ large	11	3
Grapefruit juice, unsweetened	48	8 fluid ounces	22	9
Grape jelly	52	1 Tbsp.	10	5
Grapes, fresh	53	1 cup	18	8
Green beans	★	½ cup	0	0
Green pea soup, canned	66	1 cup	41	27
Gummi confectionery, made with glucose syrup	94	1¾ ounces	36	34
Hamburger bun, white	61	½ bun (1 ounce)	15	9
Ham, lean	★■	3 ounces	0	0
Heinz® Baked Beans in tomato sauce, canned	49	½ cup	17	8

★ little or no carbs   ■ high in saturated fat

Food	GI Glucose = 100	Nominal Serving Size	Available Carbs per Serving	GL per Serving
Herbs, fresh or dried	★	2 Tbsp.	0	0
Hummus, regular	6	2 Tbsp.	5	1
ICE CREAM				
Gelati, sugar-free, chocolate	37	½ cup	14	5
Gelati, sugar-free, vanilla	39	½ cup	14	5
Ice cream, low-carb, vanilla	7	½ cup	2	0
Ice cream, low-carb, vanilla and chocolate	32	½ cup	2	1
Ice cream, low-fat, chocolate [G]	49	½ cup	14	7
Ice cream, low-fat, raspberry-ripple	55	½ cup	15	8
Ice cream, low-fat, vanilla [G]	46	½ cup	6	3
Ice cream, full-fat, average of several types	47	½ cup	13	8
Ice cream, full-fat, chocolate [G]	37	½ cup	9	4
Ice cream, full-fat, vanilla [G]	47	½ cup	15	8
Ice cream, Sara Lee®, full fat, French Vanilla	38■	½ cup	9	3
Ice cream, Sara Lee®, full fat, Ultra Chocolate	37■	½ cup	9	4
Jelly beans	78	1 ounce	28	22
Jelly, diet	★	2 Tbsp.	0	0
Kaiser bread rolls, white	73	½ roll (1 ounce)	16	12
Kavli™ Norwegian crispbread	71	1 ounce	16	12
Kidney beans, dark red, canned, drained	43	½ cup	25	7
Kidney beans, red, canned, drained	36	½ cup	17	9
Kidney beans, red, dried, boiled	28	½ cup	25	7
Kiwi fruit, fresh	53	1 medium (4 ounces)	12	6
Lamb, lean	★	4 ounces	0	0
Lean Cuisine®, French-style Chicken with Rice	36	14 ounces	72	26
Lebanese bread, white	75	1ounce	16	12
Leeks	★	½ cup	0	0

★ little or no carbs   ■ high in saturated fat

A TO Z GI TABLES

Food	GI Glucose = 100	Nominal Serving Size	Available Carbs per Serving	GL per Serving
Lemon	★	1 ounce	0	0
Lentil soup, canned	44	1 cup	21	9
Lettuce	★	1 cup	0	0
Life Savers®, peppermint	70	1 ounce	30	21
Light rye bread	68	1 ounce	14	10
Light soy milk reduced-fat, calcium-fortified	44	8 fluid ounces	17	8
Lima beans, baby, frozen, reheated	32	½ cup	30	10
Lime	★	1 ounce	0	0
Linguine pasta, thick, durum wheat, boiled	46	6 ounces	48	22
Linguine pasta, thin, durum wheat, boiled	52	6 ounces	45	23
Lychees, canned, in syrup, drained	79	½ cup	20	16
Macaroni and cheese, made from package mix, Kraft®	64■	6 ounces	51	32
Macaroni, white, plain, boiled	47	6 ounces	48	23
M&M's®, peanut	33■	1 ounce	17	6
Mango, fresh	51	½ medium (4 ounces)	17	8
Mango smoothie	32	8 fluid ounces	27	9
Maple flavored syrup	68	1 Tbsp.	22	15
Maple syrup, pure, Canadian	54	1 Tbsp.	18	10
Marmalade, 100% fruit	55	1 Tbsp.	10	6
Mars Bar®, regular	62■	2 ounces	40	25
Marshmallows, plain, white	62	1 ounce	20	12
McDonald's® Veggie Burger	59	8 ounces	55	33
Melba toast, plain	70	1 ounce	23	16
MILK				
Milk, 1 %, low-fat	32■	8 fluid ounces	12	4
Milk, 2 %, reduced-fat	30	8 fluid ounces	14	4
Milk, fat-free, skim, nonfat	32	8 fluid ounces	12	4

★ little or no carbs ■ high in saturated fat

Food	GI Glucose = 100	Nominal Serving Size	Available Carbs per Serving	GL per Serving
Milk, whole, full-fat	27	8 fluid ounces	12	4
Milk, low-fat, chocolate, with aspartame	24	8 fluid ounces	15	3
Milk, low-fat, chocolate, with sugar	34	8 fluid ounces	26	9
Condensed milk, sweetened, full-fat	61	2 fluid ounces	28	17
Rice milk, average	92	8 fluid ounces	34	31
Rice milk, calcium-riched, Vitasoy™	79	8 fluid ounces	22	17
Soy milk, full-fat, calcium fortified	36	8 fluid ounces	18	6
Soy milk, reduced-fat, calcium fortified	44	8 fluid ounces	17	8
Milk Arrowroot cookies	69■	1 ounce	18	12
Milky Bar®, plain white chocolate, Nestlé®	44■	1¾ ounces	29	13
Millet, boiled	71	¾ cup	36	25
Muesli bar, chewy, with choc. chips or fruit	54■	1 ounce	21	12
Muesli bar, crunchy with dried fruit	61	1 ounce	21	13
Mung bean noodles, cooked	33	6 ounces	45	18
Mung beans	39	½ cup	17	5
Mushrooms	★	½ cup	0	0
Muesli, untoasted, with nuts	65	2 ounces	33	21
Nectar, grape, as a sweetener [G]	52	1 Tbsp.	16	8
Nestlé® Milk Chocolate Bar	40	2 ounces	29	12
New potato, canned, microwaved 3 minutes	65	5 ounces	18	12
New potato, unpeeled and boiled 20 minutes	78	5 ounces	21	13
Nutella®, hazelnut spread	33	1 Tbsp.	12	4
Nutri-Grain™, breakfast cereal, Kellogg's®	66	½ cup	15	10
Oat Bran and honey bread	49	1 ounce	13	7

★ little or no carbs   ■ high in saturated fat

Food	GI Glucose = 100	Nominal Serving Size	Available Carbs per Serving	GL per Serving
Oat bran, unprocessed	55	2 Tbsp.	5	3
Oatmeal, instant, made with water	82	1 cup	26	17
Oatmeal, from old-fashioned rolled oats, made with water	58	1 cup	21	11
Oatmeal, from steel-cut oats, made with water	52	1 cup	22	11
Okra	★	½ cup	0	0
Onions, raw	★	½ cup	0	0
Orange, fresh	42	1 small (4 ounces)	11	5
Orange juice, unsweetened	50	8 fluid ounces	18	9
Orange, unsweetened, from concentrate	53	8 fluid ounces	18	9
Organic stoneground whole wheat sourdough bread	59	1 slice	12	7
Oysters, natural, plain	★	3 ounces	0	0
Pancakes, 6," prepared from package mix	67■	1 pancake	23	15
Parsnips	97	½ cup	12	12
PASTA				
Capellini, white, boiled	45	1 cup	45	20
Cheese tortellini, cooked	50■	6 ounces	21	10
Corn pasta, gluten-free, boiled	78	1¼ cups	42	32
Fettuccine, egg, boiled	40	1 cup	46	18
Gnocchi, cooked	68	6 ounces	48	33
Linguine, thick, durum wheat, boiled	46	1 cup	48	22
Linguine, thin, durum wheat, boiled	52	1 cup	45	23
Macaroni and cheese, Kraft®	64■	1¼ cup	51	32
Macaroni, white, durum wheat, boiled	47	1¼ cups	48	23
Macaroni, white, plain, boiled	47	1¼ cups	48	23
Ravioli, meat-filled, durum wheat flour, boiled	39■	6 ounces	38	15
Rice and corn pasta, gluten-free	76	1¼ cups	49	37
Rice pasta, brown, boiled	92	1 cup	38	35

★ little or no carbs ■ high in saturated fat

Food	GI Glucose = 100	Nominal Serving Size	Available Carbs per Serving	GL per Serving
Spaghetti, protein-enriched, boiled	27	1¼ cups	52	14
Spaghetti, white, durum wheat, cooked	44	1 cup	48	21
Spaghetti, wholewheat, cooked	42	1¼ cups	42	16
Spiral pasta, white, durum wheat, cooked	43	1¼ cups	44	19
Star Pastina, white, boiled	38	1 cup	48	18
Vermicelli, white, durum wheat, cooked	35	1 cup	44	16
Papaya, fresh	56	½ small (4 ounces)	8	5
Peaches, canned, in heavy syrup	58	½ cup	15	9
Peaches, canned, in light syrup	57	½ cup	18	9
Peaches, canned, in natural juice	45	½ cup	11	4
Peaches, fresh	42	1 medium (4 ounces)	11	5
Peanuts, roasted, salted	14	1 ¾ ounces	6	1
Pear, fresh	38	1 medium (4 ounces)	11	4
Pear halves, canned, in natural juice	44	½ cup	13	5
Pear halves, canned, in reduced-sugar syrup, SPC Lite	25	½ cup	14	4
Peas, dried, boiled	22	5 ounces	9	2
Peas, green, frozen, boiled	48	½ cup	7	3
Pecan nuts, raw	10	1 ¾ ounces	3	0
Pineapple, fresh	59	¾ cup	10	6
Pineapple juice, unsweetened	46	8 fluid ounces	34	16
Pita bread, 4" white	57	1 pita	17	10
Plum, raw	39	1 medium (4 ounces)	12	5
Polenta, boiled	68	5 ounces	13	9
Popcorn, plain, popped	72	2 cups	11	8
Pop-Tarts™, Double Chocolate	70	1 ¾ ounces	36	25
Pork	★■	3 ounces	0	0
Potato chips, plain, salted	54■	1 ¾ ounces	18	10

★ little or no carbs ■ high in saturated fat

Food	GI Glucose = 100	Nominal Serving Size	Available Carbs per Serving	GL per Serving
POTATOES				
French fries, frozen, reheated in microwave	75■	5 ounces	29	22
Potato, average, boiled	72	1 medium (5 ounces)	18	16
Potato, average, microwaved	79	1 medium (4 ounces)	18	14
Potato, russet, baked, without fat	77	1 medium (5 ounces)	30	23
Potato, instant mashed potato	85	¾ cup	20	17
Potato, new, canned, microwaved 3 minutes	65	6 small (5 ounces)	18	12
Sweet potato, baked	46	1 medium (5 ounces)	25	11
Sebago, peeled, boiled 35 mins	87	150 g	17	14
Sweet potato, baked	46	150 g	25	11
Pound cake, plain, Sara Lee	54■	1 slice (1¾ ounces)	23	12
Power Bar®, chocolate	56	65 g	42	24
Pretzels, oven-baked, traditional wheat flavor	83	1 ounce	20	16
Prune juice, natural	43	8 fluid ounces	30	13
Prunes, pitted, Sunsweet	29	2 ounces	33	10
Pudding, chocolate, instant, made from package mix, with whole milk	47	½ cup	16	7
Pudding, vanilla, instant, made from package mix, with whole milk	40	½ cup	16	6
Puffed rice cakes, white	82	25 g	21	17
Pumpkin, fresh	75	½ cup	4	3
Pumpkin soup, creamy	76	1 cup	20	15
Quinoa, organic, boiled	53	¾ cup	17	9
Radishes	★	½ cup	0	0
Raisins	64	2 ounces	44	28
Raisin bread	63	1 slice	17	11
Raspberries	★	½ cup	0	0

★ little or no carbs   ■ high in saturated fat

Food	GI Glucose = 100	Nominal Serving Size	Available Carbs per Serving	GL per Serving
Ravioli, meat-filled, durum wheat flour, boiled	39■	6 ounces	38	15
Rhubarb	★	1 cup	0	0
Rice, Arborio, risotto, white, boiled	69	¾ cup	37	24
Rice, basmati, white, boiled	58	1 cup	43	29
Rice, brown, boiled	66	1 cup	37	24
Rice, brown, quick-cooking, boiled	80	¾ cup	38	31
Rice, glutinous, white, cooked	98	¾ cup	32	31
Rice, instant, white, boiled	87	¾ cup	42	29
Rice, jasmine, white, long-grain, cooked	109	¾ cup	42	46
Rice, white, long-grain, boiled	50	¾ cup	41	23
Rice, wild, boiled	57	¾ cup	32	18
Rice bran, unprocessed	19	4 Tbsp.	14	3
Rice Krispies®, breakfast cereal, Kellogg's®	82	1¼ cups	26	22
Rice Krispie Treat™ bar, Kellogg's®	63	1 ounce	24	15
Rice cakes, puffed, white	82	1 ounce	21	17
Rice noodles, dried, boiled	61	6 ounces	39	24
Rice noodles, fresh, boiled	40	6 ounces	39	15
Rice pasta, brown, gluten-free, boiled	92	6 ounces	38	35
Rice vermicelli, dried, boiled	58	6 ounces	39	22
Rich Tea® biscuits	55■	1 ounce	19	10
Roll-Ups®, processed fruit snack	99	1 ounce	25	24
Ryvita® Country Grains crispbread	65	1 ounce	12	8
Ryvita® Original Rye crispbread	65	1 ounce	12	8
Ryvita® Sesame Rye crispbread	64	1 ounce	12	20
Salami	★■	1 ounce	0	0
Salmon, fresh, or canned in water	★	3 ounces	0	0
Sardines	★	2 ounces	0	0
Sausages, fried	28■	3 ounces	3	1
Scallions	★	1 Tbsp.	0	0
Scallops, natural, plain	★	4 ounce	0	0
Scones, plain, made from package mix	92	1 ounce	9	8

★ little or no carbs   ■ high in saturated fat

A TO Z GI TABLES

Food	GI Glucose = 100	Nominal Serving Size	Available Carbs per Serving	GL per Serving
Semolina, wheat, hot cereal, made with water	55	⅔ cup	11	6
Shallots	★	2 Tbsp.	0	0
Shellfish (shrimp, crab, lobster, etc.)	★	4 ounces	0	0
Shortbread cookies, plain	64∎	2 cookies (1 ounce)	16	10
Shredded wheat breakfast cereal	75	½ cup	20	15
Skittles®	70∎	1¾ ounces	45	32
Smoothie, banana	30	8 fluid ounces	26	8
Smoothie, mango	32	8 fluid ounces	27	9
Snowpea sprouts	★	½ cup	0	0
Soba noodles, instant, served in soup	46	6 ounces	49	22
Sourdough bread, organic, stoneground, wholewheat	59	1 slice	12	7
Sourdough rye bread	48	1 slice	12	6
Sourdough wheat bread	54	1 slice	14	8
Soybeans, canned, drained	14	½ cup	6	1
Soybeans, dried, boiled	18	½ cup	6	1
SOY MILK				
Soy milk, full-fat, calcium-fortified	36	8 fluid ounces	18	6
Soy milk, reduced-fat, calcium-fortified	44	8 fluid ounces	17	8
Soy milk, Vitasoy® Premium soy milk	18	8 fluid ounces	10	5
Soy milk, Vitasoy® Light Original	45	8 fluid ounces	10	5
Soy smoothie drink, banana, low-fat	30	8 fluid ounces	22	7
Soy smoothie drink chocolate hazelnut, low-fat	34	8 fluid ounces	25	8
Soy yogurt, fruited, 2% fat, with sugar	50	7 ounces	26	13
Special K®, regular, breakfast cereal, Kellogg's®	56	1 cup	21	11

★ little or no carbs   ∎ high in saturated fat

Food	GI Glucose = 100	Nominal Serving Size	Available Carbs per Serving	GL per Serving
Spelt multigrain bread	54	1 slice	12	7
Spinach	★	1 cup	0	0
Split pea soup, canned	60	1 cup	27	16
Sponge cake, plain, unfilled	46■	⅛ cake (2 ounces)	36	17
Squash, yellow	★	½ cup	0	0
Squid or calamari, not battered or breaded	★	4 ounces	0	0
Steak, any cut, cooked	★■	3 ounces	0	0
Stoned Wheat Thins, crackers	67	1 ounce	17	12
Strawberries, fresh	40	1 cup	3	1
Strawberry jam, 100% fruit	46	1 Tbsp.	9	4
Strawberry jam, regular, with sugar	51	1 Tbsp.	10	5
Sugar	68	2 tsp.	10	7
Raisins	56	2 ounces	45	25
Sunsweet pitted prunes	29	2 ounces	33	10
Sushi, salmon	48	3½ ounces	36	17
Sweetcorn, on the cob, boiled	48	1 medium ear	16	8
Sweetcorn, whole kernel, canned, drained	46	½ cup	14	7
Sweetened condensed full-fat milk	61■	2 ounces	28	17
Sweetened dried cranberries	64	1 ounce	29	19
Sweet potato, baked	46	1 medium (5 ounces)	25	11
Taco shells, cornmeal-based, baked	68	¾ ounces	12	8
Tofu (bean curd), plain, unsweetened	★	3½ ounces	0	0
Tomato	★	½ cup	0	0
Tomato juice, no added sugar	38	8 fluid ounces	9	4
Tomato soup, canned	45	8 fluid ounces	17	6
Tortellini, cheese, boiled	50■	6 ounces	21	10
Trout, fresh or frozen	★	4 ounces	0	0
Tuna, canned in water	★	3 ounces	0	0

★ little or no carbs   ■ high in saturated fat

A TO Z GI TABLES

Food	GI Glucose = 100	Nominal Serving Size	Available Carbs per Serving	GL per Serving
Turkey	★■	3 ounces	0	0
Turnip	★	½ cup	0	0
Twix® bar	44■	2 ounces	39	17
Udon noodles, plain	62	6 ounces	48	30
Vanilla cake made from package mix with vanilla frosting, Betty Crocker	42■	¹⁄₁₂ cake (3½ ounces)	58	24
Vanilla wafers, plain	77■	1 ounce	18	14
Veal	★	3 ounces	0	0
Veggie Burger, McDonald's	59	8 ounces	55	33
Vinegar	★	2 Tbsp.	0	0
Water crackers, plain	78	1 ounce	18	14
Watercress	★	1 cup	0	0
Watermelon, raw	76	¾ cup	6	4
Wheat, cracked, bulgur, ready to eat	48	½ cup	26	12
Whole-wheat kernels	41	1¾ ounces	34	14
Wild rice, boiled	57	¾ cup	32	18
Wonder White®, white bread	80	1 slice	15	12
Yam, peeled, boiled	37	1 medium (5 ounces)	36	13

YOGURT

Food	GI Glucose = 100	Nominal Serving Size	Available Carbs per Serving	GL per Serving
Yogurt, fat-free, with sugar, French vanilla	40	3½ ounces	27	10
Yogurt, fat-free, with sugar, mango	39	3½ ounces	25	10
Yogurt, fat-free, with sugar, strawberry	38	3½ ounces	22	8
Yogurt, fat-free, with sugar, wild berry	38	3½ ounces	22	8
Yogurt, fat-free, with sugar, average, various flavors	40	7 ounces	31	12
Yogurt, low-fat, no added sugar, vanilla, or fruit	20	7 ounces	13	3
Yogurt, low-fat, with sugar, apricot, mango, peach	26	3½ ounces	15	4

★ little or no carbs   ■ high in saturated fat

Food	GI Glucose = 100	Nominal Serving Size	Available Carbs per Serving	GL per Serving
Yogurt, low-fat, with sugar, French vanilla	26	3½ ounce	18	5
Yogurt, low-fat, with sugar, wild berry	28	3½ ounces	15	4
Yogurt, low-fat, with sugar, strawberry	28	3½ ounces	15	4
Yogurt, soy, with sugar, average, fruited	50	7 ounces	26	13
Yogurt, Yoplait, classic vanilla	36	6 ounces	33	17
Zucchini	★	½ cup	0	0

★ little or no carbs ■ high in saturated fat

Reading Sources
and References

Jenkins, D. J. A., T. M. S. Wolever, R.H., Taylor, et al. 1981.
Glycemic index of foods: A physiological basis for carbohydrate
exchange. *American Journal of Clinical Nutrition* 34: 362–6.

Salmeron, J., J. E. Manson, M. J. Stampfer, G. A. Colditz, A. L.
Wing, W. C. Willet. 1997. Dietary fiber, glycemic load and risk
of non-insulin-dependent diabetes mellitus in women. Journal of
the American Medical Association 277: 472–77.

Salmeron, J., E. B. Ascherio, G. A. Rimm, D. Colditz, D.
Spiegelman, D. J. Jenkins, M. J. Stampfer, A. A. Wing, W. C.
Willet. 1997. Dietary fiber, glycemic load and risk of NIDDM in
men. *Diabetes Care* 20: 545–50.

Liu, S., M. J. Stampfer, J. E. Manson, F. B. Ju, M. Franz, C. H.
Hennekens, W. C. Willet. 1998. A prospective study of dietary
glycemic load and risk of myocardial infarction in women. *The
Federation of American Societies for Experimental Biology Journal*
124: A260 (abstract#1517).

Frost, G., B. Keogh, D. Smith, K. Akinsanya, Ar. R. Leeds. 19954.
The effect of low glycemic carbohydrate on insulin and glucose
response in vivo and in vitro in patients with coronary heart disease. *Metabolism* 45: 669–72.

Frost, G., G. Trew, R. Margara, A. R. Leeds, A. Dornhorst. 1998.
Improvement in adipocyte insulin response to low glycemic
index diet in women at risk of cardiovascular disease. *Metabolism*
47: 1245–51.

Frost, G., A. R. Leeds, C. J. B. Dore, S. Madieros, S. A. Brading, A. Dornhorst. 1999. Glycemic index as a determinant of serum high density lipoprotein. Lancet 353: 1045–8.

Brand-Miller, J. C. 2003. Glycemic load and chronic disease. *Nutrition Review* 61 (May): S49–55.

Brand-Miller, J. C., S. Colagiuri. 1999. Evolutionary aspects of diet and insulin resistance. *World Review of Nutrition and Dietetics* 84: 74–105.

Brynes, A. E., J. Ll. Lee, R. E. Brighton, A. R. Leeds, A. Dornhorst, G. S. Frost. 2003. A low glycemic diet significantly improves the 24-h blood glucose profile in people with type 2 diabetes, as assessed using the continuous glucose MiniMed monitor. *Diabetes Care* 26(2) (Feb.): 548–9.

Foster-Powell, K., S. H. Holt, J. C. Brand-Milller. 2002. International table of glycemic index and glycemic load values: 2002. *American Journal of Clinical Nutrition* 76(1) (July): 5–56.

Hu, F. B. W. C. Willett. 2002. Optimal diets for prevention of coronary heart disease. *The Journal of the American Medical Association* 288(20) (Nov. 27): 2569–78.

Jenkins, D. J., M. Axelsen, C. W. Kendall, L. S. Augustin, V. Vuksan, U. Smith. 2000. Dietary fibre, lente carbohydrates and the insulin-resistant diseases. *British Journal of Nutrition* 83(1) (March): S157–63.

Kelly, S., G. Frost, V. Whittaker, C. Summerbell. 2004. Low glycemic index diets for coronary heart disease. *Cochrane Database of Systemic Reviews* (4) (Oct. 18): CD004467.

Leeds, A. R. 2002. Glycemic index and heart disease. *American Journal of Clinical Nutrition* 76(1)(July): 286S–9S.

Liu, S., W. C. Willett. 2002. Dietary glycemic load and atherothrombotic risk. *Current Atheroscler Reports* 4(6) (Nov.): 454–61.

McKeown, N. M., J. B. Meigs, S. Liu, E. Saltzman, P. W. Wilson, P. F. Jacques. 2004. Carbohydrate nutrition, insulin resistance, and the prevalence of the metabolic syndrome in the Framingham Offspring Cohort. *Diabetes Care* 27(2) (Feb.): 538–46.

McMillan-Price, J., J. Brand-Miller. 2004. Dietary approaches to overweight and obesity. *The American Journal of Clinical Dermatology* 22(4) (Jul.–Aug.): 310–4.

READING SOURCES AND REFERENCES

Patel, V. C., R. D. Aldridge, A. Leeds, A. Dornhorst, G. S. Frost. 2004. Retrospective analysis of the impact of a low glycemic index diet on hospital stay following coronary artery bypass grafting: A hypothesis. *Journal of Human Nutrition and Dietetics* 17(3) (June): 241–7.

Skurk, T., H. Hauner. 2004. Obesity and impaired fibrinolysis: Role of adipose production of plasminogen activator inhibitor-1. *International Journal of Obesity and Related Metabolic Disorders* 28(11) (Nov.): 1357–64.

Trayhurn, P., I. S. Wood. 2004. Adipokines: Inflammation and the pleiotropic role of white adipose tissue. *British Journal of Nutrition* 92(3) (Sept.): 347–55.

Wilkin, T. J., L. D. Voss. 2004. Metabolic syndrome: Maladaptation to a modern world. *Journal of the Royal Society of Medicine* 97(11) (Nov.): 511–20.

About the authors

Professor Jennie Brand-Miller is Professor of Human Nutrition in the Human Nutrition Unit, School of Molecular and Microbial Biosciences at the University of Sydney, and President of the Nutrition Society of Australia. She has taught postgraduate students of nutrition and dietetics at the University of Sydney for over 25 years and currently leads a team of 12 research scientists.

Kaye Foster-Powell is an accredited practicing dietitian with extensive experience in diabetes management. A graduate of the University of Sydney (B.Sc., Master of Nutrition & Dietetics), she has conducted research into the glycemic index of foods and its practical applications over the last 15 years. Currently she is the senior dietitian with Sydney West Diabetes Service and provides consulting on all aspects of the glycemic index.

Dr. Anthony Leeds is Senior Lecturer in the Department of Nutrition & Dietetics at King's College, London. He graduated in medicine from the Middlesex Hospital Medical

School, London, in 1971. He conducts research on carbohydrate and dietary fiber in relation to heart disease, obesity, and diabetes and continues part-time medical practice.
In 1999 he was elected a Fellow of the Institute of Biology.

Acknowledgments

We are indebted to our dietitian colleagues who generously gave up their time to help us with the Asian and Mediterranean meal ideas for this edition. We would like to thank Johanna Burani for the Mediterranean meal ideas; Linda Cumines for the Chinese meal ideas; Effie Houvardis for the Middle Eastern and South-East Asian meal ideas; and Sangita Nayak for the Indian meal ideas.

The totally tireless production team at Hachette Livre Australia always make it easy for us and graciously squeeze deadlines to suit our schedules. We would particularly like to thank Fiona Hazard (Publishing and Production Director) and Anna Waddington (Production Editor) for making it all happen, and our editor, Jacquie Brown, for her patience and meticulous attention to detail.

A special thank you to Fiona Atkinson and the dedicated GI testing team at the University of Sydney—Anna, Marian and Kai Lyn—and all our cheerful, well-fed volunteers. Thank you also to Associate Professor Gareth Denyer for his invaluable help with the GI database.

ACKNOWLEDGMENTS

And of course we wouldn't have made it through so many late nights and working weekends without the loving support of our husbands, John Miller and Jonathan Powell. Thank you.

Index

abdominal obesity
  metabolic syndrome from, 1,
    20, 21
  waist measurement, 21–22,
    25–26, 32
acidity and GI value, 45
aerobic exercise, 26
alcohol, moderation with, 36,
  76–77
American Dietetic Association, 62
anthocyanins, 69
antioxidants, 69
apple body shape, 20–21
arteries, 9, 14–16, 16
Asian-style diets
  breakfasts, 106–7
  desserts, 111–12
  dinners, 109–11
  eating out, 105
  lunches, 107–8
  overview, 102–4
  snacks, 112–13
atherosclerosis, 1–2, 9
A to Z GI tables, 121–38

Barbecued Beef Kebabs, 87
beans, ideas for using, 67, 68
beverages, 85
BGL. *See* blood glucose level
blood clots (thrombosis), 9, 10, 68
blood glucose level (BGL)
  and GI value of foods, 43
  and heart disease, 2, 14–16
  high-to-low swings in, 33
  as insulin resistance indicator, 32
  and low-GI foods, 41, 45–47
BMI (body mass index), 50–51
body shape, apple or pear, 20–21
breakfasts
  Asian-style, 106–7
  basics, 81
  Mediterranean-style, 97, 98
  multiethnic suggestions for,
    86–92, 93
butter, fats in, 36

calcium, 78–80
calories in heart-healthy menu
  suggestions, 84

candy substitutes, 55
carbohydrates
  in heart-healthy menu
    suggestions, 84
  insulin level and burning of, 32
  and insulin production, 30–31
  overview, 42
  rate of digestion, 48–49
  relationship to GI diet, 51–52
cardiovascular event frequency, 1,
  29–30
cardiovascular fitness, improving,
  26
changing eating habits, 61–62
chicken, 53, 60, 80
chickpeas, 67
Chinese diet, 51. *See also* Asian-
  style diets
Chinese meal suggestions, 106,
  107, 109, 111, 112
cholesterol, 16–17, 66, 81. *See
  also* HDL cholesterol
cod liver oil and cholesterol levels,
  37
Couscous with Chickpeas, 97
C-reactive protein (CRP), 12, 19
Creamy Pasta, 90
CRP (C-reactive protein), 12, 19

dairy products, 53, 59, 68, 78–80
desserts
  Asian-style, 111–12
  low-GI, 94–95
  Mediterranean-style, 97,
    100–101
diabetes (impaired glucose
  tolerance), 1, 14–16, 30–31, 48
diet. *See also* fat in foods
  dieters' problems with, 21, 22,
    23–24, 54
  and fibrinolysis effectiveness,
    10

low-carb, effects of, 23–24
  and weight, 22
Dietary Guidelines for Americans
  (2005), 76
dietitians, registered, 62
dinners
  Asian-style, 109–11
  basics, 82
  Mediterranean-style, 97, 99–100
  multiethnic suggestions for, 92,
    93–94
dinner recipes
  Barbecued Beef Kebabs, 87
  Couscous with Chickpeas, 97
  Creamy Pasta, 90
  Minestrone Soup, 86
  Moroccan Lamb and Spicy
    Rice, 91
  Salmon Cakes, 89
  Vegetarian Pizza, 88
doctors
  identifying cardiovascular
    disease, 30
  for metabolic indicator tests,
    14, 16, 18
  before starting exercise routine,
    29
  treatments for heart disease,
    10–11

eating habits, tips for changing,
  61–62
eating out Asian-style, 105
eatright.org, 62
eggs, 36, 53, 81
essential fatty acids, 73
ethnic origin and insulin
  resistance, 32
exercise, 10, 24–29

family history (genes), 10, 16–17,
  32, 34–35

INDEX

fat in foods
  fat counter, 58–61
  fat storage process, 33
  fatty plaque from, 15
  and GI value, 45
  low-fat versus regular milk, 79
  meats, 59, 73
  saturated fats, 16–17, 32, 36, 73–74
  unsaturated fats, 37, 73–74, 77, 85, 96
fiber, 45, 65–66
fibrinolysis, 10
fish, mercury in, 72–73
fish and seafood, 53, 60, 71–73
fitness, exercise program and, 28
Food and Drug Administration, 72–73
free radicals, 15
French fry substitutes, 55
fruits and vegetables, 69–71

genetic factors, 10, 16–17, 32, 34–35
GI. See glycemic index
GI Symbol Program, 119
GL (glycemic load), 53–54, 117–20
glucose, 33, 42. See also blood glucose level
glycemic index (GI)
  benefits of eating low on the list, 46, 48–49
  definition of, 43
  difficulty of measuring values, 52–53
  factors influencing GI value of foods, 43–45
  overview, 2, 3, 34–35
glycemic index tables, 121–38
glycemic load (GL), 53–54, 117–20
Greece, 96. See also
  Mediterranean-style diets

Harvard University "Nurses Study," 50–51
HDL (high-density lipoprotein) cholesterol
  correlation with glycemic load, 48–49
  high BGL versus, 15
  low level as metabolic syndrome risk factor, 48
  overview, 17, 18, 48
  in soy foods, 68
heart disease
  insulin-resistance and, 32–33
  long-term prevention of, 48–49
  research on role of GI in, 50–51
  testing your knowledge about, 35–37
  treatments for, 10–11
heart disease risk factors. See also metabolic syndrome
  blood glucose level, 2, 14–16
  C-reactive protein, 19
  high blood cholesterol, 16–18
  high blood pressure, 13–14
  overview, 11–12
  overweight and obesity, 19–24
  saturated fats, 16–17, 32, 36, 73–74
  sedentary lifestyle, 24
  smoking, 12–13
heart healthy diet. See also low-GI diet
  alcohol, moderating amount of, 36, 76–77
  chicken, skinless, 80
  dairy, low-fat, 78–80
  fats, replacing bad with good, 73–74
  fish and seafood, 71–73
  fruits and vegetables, 69–71
  legumes, 67–68
  nuts, including, 77–78

heart healthy diet (*continued*)
  red meats, lean, 80
  salt intake, minimizing, 75
  soy products, calcium-enriched, 79
  whole grain breads and cereals, 65–66
heat production from exercise, 25
heredity. *See* genetic factors
high amylose to amylopectin ratio and GI value, 44
high blood cholesterol, 16–18
high blood pressure, 1, 13–14
high cholesterol foods, 18
high-density lipoprotein. *See* HDL cholesterol
high-GI diet, detrimental chain reaction from, 48
high-GI foods, 2, 32–33
hypertension, 1, 13–14

IDF (International Diabetes Federation), 21, 30
impaired glucose tolerance. *See* diabetes; pre-diabetes
incidental activity, increasing amount of, 27
incremental weight gain, 24
Indian diet, 102. *See also* Asian-style diets
Indian meal suggestions, 106–7, 108, 110–11, 112, 113
inflammation, definition of, 19
insensitivity to insulin. *See* insulin resistance syndrome
insoluble fiber, 66
insulin, 30–31, 42, 48
insulin levels, 15, 31–32, 48
insulin resistance syndrome. *See also* metabolic syndrome
  and BMI, 50–51
  ethnic origin and, 32

overview, 1, 29, 31–33
  relationship to metabolic syndrome, 30
insulin-resistance tests, 30
insulin sensitivity, 34–35, 48–49, 50–51, 65
International Diabetes Federation (IDF), 21, 30
isoflavones, 68

lactose, 78–79
lactose intolerance, 79–80
LDL (low-density lipoprotein) cholesterol, 17, 68
legumes, 67–68
lentils, 67
lifestyle factors, 16–17, 24–29. *See also* abdominal obesity
low-carb diet, 23–24, 54
low-density lipoprotein (LDL) cholesterol, 17, 68
low-GI diet. *See also* heart healthy diet
  achieving an effective reduction, 56–58
  advantages for dieters, 22, 24
  benefits of, 2–4, 41, 49
  the non-isolation principle, 52, 85
  overview, 48, 84–85
  portion size considerations, 54, 83
  pre-surgery research on, 34
  this for that method of utilizing, 51, 54–56
  and weight loss, 21–22
low-GI meals. *See* breakfasts; dinners; lunches; salads; snack foods
low-sodium, meaning of, 75
lunches
  Asian-style, 107–8
  basics, 82

Mediterranean-style, 97, 98–99
multiethnic suggestions for, 86–91, 93
Omelet, 92

margarine, fats in, 36
meat
 benefits of lean, red, 80
 fat content of, 59, 73
 GI not applicable to, 53
 salt in, 75
Mediterranean-style diets
 meal suggestions, 97–101
 overview, 96–97
menus
 Asian-style, 104
 Mediterranean-style, 97
 a week of heart-healthy, low-GI eating, 84–85
mercury in fish, 72–73
metabolic rate, effect of exercise, 25
metabolic syndrome. See also insulin resistance syndrome
 features contributing to, 1–2
 IDF criteria for defining, 21, 30
 obesity and, 1, 20, 21–22, 25–26, 32
 overview, 29–31
 prevention of, 10
 risk factors, 21, 30, 48
Minestrone Soup, 86
monounsaturated fats, 37, 73–74, 96
Moroccan Lamb and Spicy Rice, 91

National Institute on Alcohol Abuse and Alcoholism, 77
National Network of Tobacco Cessation Quitlines, 13

Nurses Study at Harvard School of Public Health, 50–51
nuts, 37, 77–78

obesity, 30, 50. See also abdominal obesity
olive oil, 36
omega-3 fatty acids, 71–73
Omelet, 92
optimum health. See also low-GI diet
 monitor metabolic indicators, 14–16, 18
 quitting smoking, 12–13
 recommended fat intake per day, 58–61
 slow rate of carbohydrate digestion, 48–51
 this for that method of substitution, 51, 54–56

palpitations, 10
pancreas, 30–31
particle size and GI value, 44
pasta al dente as low GI, 44
pasta is fattening myth, 37
pear body shape, 20–21
personal trainers, 28–29
physical entrapment of nutrients and GI value, 44
plant sterols, 16–17
polyunsaturated fats, 37, 73–74, 96
pork, fat content of, 60
portion size considerations, 54, 83
potatoes
 combining with corn, 52, 56
 high GI rating of, 46–47
 reducing glycemic response to, 70–71
 restricting, 54, 56
prediabetes (impaired glucose tolerance), 1, 14–16

primary prevention, 10
processed foods, 24
proteins, 52, 53

rate of carbohydrate digestion, 2, 3, 45–51
refined foods, 24
registered dietitians (RDs), 62
resources
  for alcohol abuse prevention, 77
  eatright.org, 62
  glycemicindex.com, 43
  glycemic index research, 120
  reading material, 139–41
  for smoking cessation, 13
restricted blood flow. See atherosclerosis
rice, 103–4
risk factors. See also heart disease risk factors
  for insulin resistance, 31–32
  for metabolic syndrome, 21, 30
  for thrombosis, 10
roughage, 66

salads, simple combos for, 94
Salmon Cakes, 89
salt intake, 75
saturated fats, 16–17, 32, 36, 73–74
seafood and fish, 71–73
secondary prevention, 10
sedentary lifestyle, 24
smoking and heart disease, 12–13
snack foods
  Asian-style, 112–13
  fat content of, 60
  Mediterranean-style, 97, 101
  multiethnic suggestions for heart healthy, 86–92
  suggestions for heart healthy, 95

soluble fibers, 66
sources of information. See resources
Southeast Asian meal suggestions, 106, 107–8, 109–10, 111–12, 113. See also Asian-style diets
soybeans and soy products, 67–68, 79
starch gelatinization, 44
sugar, 45, 56
Syndrome X, 1, 29. See also metabolic syndrome

this for that method of substitution, 51, 54–56
thrombosis (blood clot), 9, 10, 68
tips for changing eating habits, 61–62
treats, 85
triglycerides, 17, 33, 48
type 2 diabetes, high-GI foods leading to, 30–31

unsaturated fats, 37, 73–74, 77, 84, 96

vegetables and fruits, 69–71, 94
Vegetarian Pizza, 88
viscosity of fiber and GI value, 45
vitamin A, 37, 69

waist measurement, 21–22, 25–26, 32
walking, value of, 27–28
weight, 17, 28, 30, 50. See also abdominal obesity
white bread substitutes, 55, 65–66
whole grain breads and cereals, 65–66